Personal Experience of a Physician

John Ellis

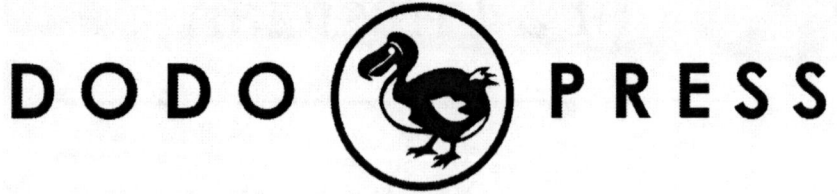

PERSONAL EXPERIENCE OF A PHYSICIAN,

WITH

AN APPEAL TO THE MEDICAL AND CLERICAL PROFESSIONS;

AND

AN APPENDIX,

A REVIEW OF "CHRIST AND THE TEMPERANCE QUESTION" IN
THE CHRISTIAN UNION.

BY

JOHN ELLIS, M.D.

CONTENTS.

CHAPTER I.
PERSONAL MEDICAL EXPERIENCE OF A PHYSICIAN.

CHAPTER II.
WHY EVERY PHYSICIAN SHOULD EXAMINE HOMOEOPATHY.

CHAPTER III.
DANGERS THAT RESULT FROM THE ALLOPATHIC TREATMENT OF DISEASES.

CHAPTER IV.
PERSONAL RELIGIOUS EXPERIENCE OF A PHYSICIAN.

CHAPTER V.
THE DAWN OF A NEW DISPENSATION.

CHAPTER VI.
A NEW DAY TO OUR EARTH.

CHAPTER VII.
THE WANTS OF THE CHRISTIAN CHURCH.

CHAPTER VIII.
RESTRAINING AND CURING SPIRITUAL AND NATURAL DISEASES.

CHAPTER IX.
PERSONAL EXPERIENCE CONTINUED AND EFFORTS.

CHAPTER X.
FINAL APPEAL TO THE CLERGY.

ADDENDUM.
A REVIEW OF "CHRIST AND THE TEMPERANCE QUESTION," IN THE "CHRISTIAN UNION."

Personal Experience of a Physician

CHAPTER I.

PERSONAL MEDICAL EXPERIENCE OF A PHYSICIAN.

We all admit that every one who attempts to act as a physician, should strive to qualify himself, or herself, for the work by obtaining the best education which our medical schools afford; for to physicians are intrusted, not simply the property or money, but the very lives of their fellow-citizens. As the responsibility is great, so the duty of preparing one's self before commencing practice, and of keeping fully abreast of all new and valuable discoveries in the art of healing, is equally great. A physician should not be led blindly by his teachers and prominent medical writers, and so strongly confirm himself in the theories and views which they proclaim that he cannot, without prejudice, examine new views and theories with due care. It has been said that when Harvey discovered the true course of the circulation of the blood, there was not a single professor in the medical colleges of England over fifty years of age, who ever believed "the heresy, " as his discovery was called. However this may have been, it is certain that professors and prominent medical writers are not always the first to see and recognize the truth, even when it is clearly presented to their notice.

A native of western Massachusetts, I studied medicine with an intelligent and worthy physician in my native town, and attended two and one-half courses of medical lectures at the Berkshire Medical College, at Pittsfield, Mass., and graduated in 1841; and during the following winter I attended the Medical College at Albany, N. Y., devoting a large portion of my time to dissecting. After finishing at Albany, I visited various places in western and central Massachusetts, and operated on eyes for strabismus or cross-eyes, —an operation which had then been recently introduced for that deformity; after which I settled at Chesterfield (Mass.), and commenced practicing medicine, where I remained about one year.

One day I visited Northampton, and, calling on a physician with whom I was acquainted, I found upon his table a homoeopathic book. "Why, " I exclaimed with astonishment, "you are not studying homoeopathy, are you? " "Yes, " he replied, "I am studying it, and trying the remedies cautiously; " and he went on to describe cases which he had treated satisfactorily by the use of the remedies, and among them a case of pleurisy and one of intermittent fever, and he wound up by saying: "Now, if you will go down the street to a bookstore and purchase 'Hull's Jahr, ' in two volumes, I will give you half a dozen homoeopathic remedies, and you can try them for yourself. "

Here was a dilemma. Never until that hour had I ever heard homoeopathy spoken of, by either a medical professor or one of my professional brethren, except with contempt and ridicule. "But, " I said to myself, "if there is any truth in homoeopathy I ought to know it, and I cannot treat this physician's testimony with contempt; and it is a duty which I owe to my fellow-men, and especially to my patients, to investigate the new system carefully. " I immediately went and purchased the books, and he give me six bottles of medicine, and I took them back with me to Chesterfield. I remember making but one Homoeopathic prescription before leaving Chesterfield, and that was for a case of uterine hemorrhage, which I had treated unsuccessfully for some time with allopathic remedies. I looked over my Homoeopathic books carefully and found that China (cinchona) was indicated. As that remedy was not among the bottles of medicated pellets which my medical friend had given me, I directed that one drop of the ordinary tincture of Peruvian bark should be dropped into a glass of water, and that, after stirring it well, one teaspoonful of the solution thus made should be given three or four times a day. The patient commenced improving immediately, and was soon well.

Soon after that I removed to Grand Rapids, Michigan, and commenced anew the practice of medicine. I then had neither the knowledge nor the faith in homoeopathy which I thought would justify me in treating any serious case of disease with homoeopathic remedies; but I did not neglect to study the new books. One day, a friend of my younger days, who was residing at Grand Haven, came into my office and said that he had been suffering from the toothache for several days, and that he did not like to have the tooth extracted, and he wanted to know if I could do anything for it without extracting it. I told him that I had recently obtained some homoeopathic books and remedies, and that I had noticed that remedies were spoken of for toothache. So I looked over my books and selected Belladonna as the remedy suitable in his case, and gave him a dose of it and other doses to take with him if he needed them. We talked in the office for a short time, and then we walked up to the hotel where he was stopping; as we entered, he stood still a moment and remarked: "Well, my tooth does not ache as severely as it did. " I saw him weeks afterward, and he told me that he had not had the toothache from the hour he took the medicine.

Away in that new place, then a village of about one thousand inhabitants, with no homoeopathic physician within a hundred miles of me, I commenced cautiously the use of the new remedies; first in mild cases of disease, and in cases where Allopathic treatment failed to produce the desired effect. Among the first of the serious cases where I used the remedies was a case of pneumonia. A young man had been very sick with that disease for many days. I had resorted vigorously to the antiphlogistic treatment then in vogue; a consulting physician was called, and at last we told the family that our patient could not live until the next morning. I then said to the consulting physician: "I have some homoeopathic remedies; suppose we try them? " His reply was: "It does not make any difference what you try; he will not live until morning. " Under such circumstances I felt that I was justified in trying the new remedies. I accordingly dissolved a few pellets of Aconite in a glass of water, and of Bryonia alb. in another glass of water, and directed that a teaspoonful of the solution of Aconite should be given once an hour for five hours, and that a similar dose of Bryonia be given instead of Aconite every sixth hour. I sat down by his bedside and watched his case for two hours. At the end of that period I found that his pulse was five beats less frequent in a minute, and that his breathing was a little easier. The next morning all of his dangerous symptoms had disappeared, and in a reasonable period of time he was restored to health. I talked with the consulting physician about his unexpected recovery, and we were, disposed to think that we had made a false prognosis, and that he would have recovered any way. Still, the case made some impression on me; so that in the next case of pneumonia to which I was called, I resolved to try the same remedies in the same way. The patient was a man about forty years of age. Under the action of the Aconite and Bryonia the patient about held his own, neither gaining nor losing very perceptibly for about three days. At the end of that period I became alarmed, and felt that if the patient were to die I should be guilty of the crime of manslaughter. I discontinued the treatment, and resorted to the then regular antiphlogistic treatment; the patient immediately began to get worse, and at the end of three days more he was a very sick man. I then came to the conclusion that my patient had done much better under the homoeopathic treatment than he had under the Allopathic, and I discontinued the latter and returned to the former, giving the Aconite and Bryonia. The patient ceased to grow worse; he held his own for two or three days, then he began to improve, and was soon restored to health. From that day to this I have never bled a patient suffering from either pneumonia or pleurisy, neither have I applied a blister, or given a cathartic, or an Allopathic dose of tartar emetic, or an opiate, or any form of alcoholic or fermented drinks, either during the continuance of the above-named diseases or during convalescence; nor have I ever regretted, in a single instance, not having done so.

During the fall of the year we had many cases of dysentery which were very obstinate, continuing one or two weeks or longer, attended by a fever approaching a typhoid character. I found the Allopathic treatment unsatisfactory, as there were quite a number of deaths. So I consulted my homoeopathic books and concluded to try the remedies; but at that time I had only the six carefully prepared remedies given me by the physician in Northampton, and I found that I needed some other remedies; so for Arsenicum I used a drop of Fowler's solution of arsenic in a glassful of water, giving a teaspoonful of the solution thus prepared for a dose, and I also used the tincture of Colocynth and other remedies in the same manner. Even with the help of such crude remedies I found that I could generally control the disease far more speedily and with greater certainty and safety than by Allopathic treatment.

I was called to attend a young man who, while stooping over to set a trap in the woods, was mistaken for a bear by a comrade who was hunting with him, and shot through the neck. To restrain secondary hemorrhage I was obliged, in order to save the life of my patient, to ligature both carotid arteries at the interval of only four and one-half days, which, at that time, had never been done successfully at an interval of less than twelve months between the operations. My patient did not suffer from head symptoms, as I was fearful he would, but his lungs became seriously congested. I resorted to the Allopathic treatment without affording any relief; and, as he was steadily getting worse, I consulted my homoeopathic works and gave him Aconite, a drop of the tincture in a glass of water; of the solution thus made I directed a teaspoonful to be given every hour; this gave prompt relief to the active symptoms of congestion. For a cough which remained I gave a few doses of belladonna prepared in the same manner, and all of the symptoms soon disappeared. I reported this case to the New York Journal of Medicine, and it was transferred, even to the homoeopathic prescriptions, to the American edition of Velpeau's great work on surgery.

Personal Experience of a Physician

I found when I went to Grand Rapids that the intermittent, remittent, and pernicious fevers, which prevailed in that place and in the surrounding country, were generally treated by the resident physicians with mercurial or other cathartic remedies, followed or accompanied by Quinine and brandy or fermented drinks containing Alcohol, and opiates where they were supposed to be necessary. As I began to look into homoeopathy, I first prescribed Ipecac for the vomiting which sometimes attended these fevers, one drop of the tincture in a glass of water, and giving a teaspoonful from the glass for a dose. For watery diarrhoeas I gave Fowler's solution of Arsenic in the same manner, and in both instances generally with very satisfactory results. As my confidence in the homoeopathic treatment of diseases increased, I sent to New York and obtained an assortment of the remedies and more books, and was then much better prepared to prescribe successfully. I soon found that by their use I could dispense with cathartic remedies and thus avoid the danger of causing a medicinal irritation of the bowels, which it is sometimes difficult to control. I also found that I could do much better without Alcohol in any form, in the treatment of these fevers, than with it; and I soon ceased to use brandy, wine, beer, etc.

As to Quinine, that remedy will unquestionably interrupt the paroxysms of intermittent and remittent fevers promptly if it is given at the proper time and in suitable doses; and, if the attack is the first the patient has ever had, a return of the disease may at least sometimes be prevented by giving once a week in two or three doses, at an interval of twelve hours, about the quantity which would be required to interrupt the disease in the first instance. These doses should be given the day before the disease is expected to return. I found it much better to give about two large doses of quinine than to give the same quantity in 1 or 2 grain doses. I reported the results of my experiments and observations in the use of Quinine at Grand Rapids to the *New York Journal of Medicine* (allopathic). In all instances where life is in danger from a return of a paroxysm of intermittent or remittent fever, the patient can be rescued from immediate danger by giving Quinine in doses sufficient to prevent a return of the paroxysm. In all other cases, and perhaps even in such, we can rely safely on homoeopathic remedies in minute doses. Quinine in Allopathic doses will rarely cure the disease, excepting, it may be, as named above, in a first attack. If the patient has ever had more than one or two attacks, it is almost sure to return again and again for two seasons, complicated with symptoms caused by the remedy, in spite of Allopathic doses of quinine; whereas by treating the patient homoeopathically, except in old cases, you will not suddenly interrupt the paroxysms, for they may continue one or two weeks, or even a few days longer, but when they cease there is generally the end of the disease, and the patient speedily regains his ordinary state of health instead of lingering along with frequent returns of the disease for generally two seasons, as he does when quinine is used. Old cases of intermittent fever are frequently cured promptly by infinitesimal doses of homoeopathic remedies. I have never seen Allopathic doses of Quinine do any good in typhoid fevers. And, as to the use of cathartics, from my observation I soon became satisfied that a vast number of lives have been lost by their use in cases of remittent and typhoid fevers, the tendency to irritation of the mucous membrane, which exists especially in the latter disease, being often fatally aggravated by cathartic remedies.

I found the prejudice so strong against homoeopathy when I commenced my investigations, that I generally said nothing about the kind of remedies I was using, and sometimes disguised the remedies by mixing with sugar or pulverized liquorice root, or by mixing or dissolving them in water.

I have given the above details to show how carefully and patiently, step by step, I commenced my investigations, and watched the action of remedies when given in accordance with the Homoeopathic law of cure, and compared the results with the results which followed the use of Allopathic remedies.

I remained at Grand Rapids two years. During that period I gradually substituted the Homoeopathic treatment of diseases for the Allopathic, as fast as I found I could cure the various diseases which came under my observation with more safety and certainty by the former method of treatment than by the latter.

Now I ask the intelligent, conscientious, and philanthropic reader, Did I do right or did I do wrong in thus investigating homoeopathy and using cautiously the remedies for the cure of the sick, as I found them more efficacious and safe than the remedies which I had been taught to use and had used previously? If it was my duty to thus critically examine the new method of treatment, when my attention was seriously called to it, and to cautiously try the remedies on the sick, is it not clearly the duty of every Allopathic physician in our land to do the same? To thus earnestly call the attention of physicians of every school to the importance of investigating homoeopathy, and carefully using the remedies for the cure of the sick, and to entreat them not to stop and be satisfied with crude doses, such as drop doses of tinctures and the first, second or third dilutions or triturations of remedies, as some have done, is my sole object in writing these pages. The most decided and satisfactory cures which I have ever witnessed have been effected by the thirtieth and two hundredth dilutions. But, according to my experience, it is not well to confine one's self absolutely to either high or low dilutions, as some have done; but if you are satisfied that you have selected the right remedy, instead of changing the remedy when you do not see relief from its use, change the dilution from low to high or high to low, as the case may be. I could detail many cases to show the importance of doing this. No physician should labor specially to sustain either a theory or preconceived ideas, but to cure his patients promptly. The health and lives of our fellow-beings are too important to be trifled with.

During the early years of my practice of homoeopathy I was called to see a young man recently attacked with "epileptic fits. " As he was going immediately to New York, with his sister, I advised them to call on the late Dr. John F. Gray, with whom I became acquainted during my first visit to New York. On reaching New York they called on Dr. Gray, and the young man remained under his treatment for several weeks. Of Dr. Gray's treatment of this patient, so far as remedies were concerned, I know only of a single remedy which he gave, which was Nitrate of silver, which I understood was given in a somewhat crude form, and not even in a low centesimal dilution. The young man, finding little or no benefit from the treatment, went to his home in Georgia, after which I received a letter stating that he had not been essentially benefited by Dr. Gray's treatment, and requesting me to prescribe for him. In response I sent him the 30th dilution of Nux vomica, which he took and soon recovered from the disease, and never had any return of the paroxysms. Dr. Gray was a low dilutionist.

On the other hand, during my second or third visit to New York I called on Dr. Edward Bayard, who was a high dilutionist. I found him in poor health. He had been suffering, as he told me, for some time from a subacute irritation of the mucous membrane of the bowels, with loose passages, and some febrile excitement. He asked me to prescribe for him. After a careful inquiry as to existing symptoms I said to him, "Mercurius vivus ought to cure you. " He replied that he had taken it repeatedly without the slightest effect. I asked him what dilution of this remedy he had taken. He replied that he had taken the 30th and 200th dilutions. I suggested that he should take the 3d trituration. "Why, " he exclaimed, "I have not prescribed the 3d trituration of mercury for many years, and I do not know as I have any in my office. " But, on looking around, he found a bottle of the second centesimal trituration; and I said to him: "That will answer. You can take a dose of that now [which he did] and repeat it three or four times between now and to-morrow night, after which take a dose of the 30th or 200th dilution of sulphur. " The next time I saw him he told me that my prescription cured him promptly.

That the careful treatment of diseases by the use of low dilutions of Homoeopathic remedies, when compared with the Allopathic treatment, is wonderfully successful I well know; for it was by the success which attended the use of the low dilutions that I was led into the new practice, as thousands of other graduates of allopathic colleges have been. Still, I know very well by experience that the low dilutionists, in a very large number of cases, fail to cure patients promptly, and in many cases fail to cure them at all when they could cure them promptly by the use of the high dilutions, often by the very same remedy which they have been using. I was called to see a patient suffering from puerperal anaemia, with "nursing sore mouth. " She was greatly exhausted; her stomach, which was very acid, would retain very little nourishment. She had been under Allopathic treatment for some time without experiencing any relief. I gave her a low dilution of Pulsatilla, which afforded her no relief. Then I selected other remedies, from which she derived no benefit. After that I gave her the 200th dilution of Pulsatilla, the first dose of which produced, as she declared, a change for the better within an hour, and she rapidly recovered under its use. A lady who had for two winters been sent to Florida by her Allopathic physician for a severe cough, attended by the physical signs of induration of the summit of one of her lungs, called on me early in the fall, saying that her physician advised her to go again to Florida, but that she did not like to go, and wanted me to prescribe for her. After examining her symptoms carefully I gave her a single dose of Sulphur, 200th dilution; at the end of a week she was better, at the end of another week much better, and at the end of the third week she had but few symptoms remaining, for which I gave only one dose of Arsenicum, 200th, which completed the cure.

Personal Experience of a Physician

Having practiced medicine for two years at Grand Rapids, I spent a winter East and visited New York, making the Acquaintance of Homoeopathic physicians, and conversing with them about the new system of treating disease, attending medical lectures and clinics at the two Allopathic colleges. I remember very well attending a clinic at the College of Physicians and Surgeons, held by the late Prof. Willard Parker, when a little child was brought in suffering from whooping cough. Prof. Parker, looking around upon the students, said: "Here, gentlemen, is a case of disease which, like the small-pox, measles, and scarlet fever, runs a definite course; if you will let the patients alone they will generally get well, but if you commence dosing them you will often bring on complications and they will die. " This statement, coming from a medical man of his prominence, surely was worthy of consideration.

After spending the winter at the East I went to Detroit, Mich., and opened an office in connection with Dr. P. M. Wheaton. I practiced in Detroit for fifteen years, excepting that during the last six years of that time I spent a part of each year at Cleveland, giving a course of lectures on the Theory and Practice of Medicine at the Western Homoeopathic Medical College, of Cleveland, Ohio.

When I went to Detroit the prejudice against homoeopathy was very strong, especially among physicians. An attempt was made to pass a bill through the Legislature of Michigan which would virtually prohibit the practice in the State. The bill passed the Senate, but, owing to the prompt action of the friends of homoeopathy in exposing the design of the advocates of the bill, it was defeated in the House of Representatives. The presence of the Asiatic cholera in 1849 in the city, and the success which attended the homoeopathic treatment of that disease, was instrumental in calling the attention of large numbers of the most intelligent and influential citizens to the new practice and establishing it upon a firm basis. When the disease first appeared in the city, we furnished the families which we were accustomed to attend, and all others who desired them, with Veratrum album and Cuprum metallicum, which had been earnestly recommended by Homoeopathic physicians elsewhere, who had had experience in treating the disease, as preventive remedies, a dose or two of each to be taken daily. As a result, very few among the families which we were accustomed to attend were attacked with the disease, and in such cases as occurred the disease was generally readily controlled. As a rule, the most troublesome cases which we had to treat were those in which Opium or morphine in some form had been administered before we were called. In such cases it was exceedingly difficult to get a satisfactory response from our remedies, however carefully we selected them.

The Asiatic cholera is a violent disease and rapid in its progress, and if severe cases of this disease are to be treated successfully, it must be by remedies which are prompt in their action. It is here that homoeopathic remedies show their superiority over all other remedies or methods of treatment, for they act upon the diseased organs in the direction of the disease, and thus excite a prompt reaction. Homoeopathic remedies, when properly used, do not benumb, nor do they seriously aggravate existing diseased action; and they neither cause diseased action in well organs, nor reduce the quantity of blood, nor lessen the vitality of the organism and the ability to react against the encroachment of diseased action, as does the allopathic treatment; and, consequently, if a patient dies the physician and his friends have the consolation, at least, of knowing that he did not die from the treatment.

I well remember, while practicing in Detroit, attending a prominent citizen, a lawyer, who had a severe attack of pneumonia; and, while recovering from it, he went one night into a cold room to sleep, and this brought on a relapse which involved both lungs, and my patient became very sick. One day on visiting him I found an Allopathic physician sitting by his bedside. I was told that he simply called as a friend. As I entered he arose and walked out into the hall. I followed him, and asked him what he thought of my patient. He replied very promptly: "He will die! he will die, sir!! He ought to have been bled, blistered, and physicked long ago, but it is too late now. " I replied: "He will not die, sir, for the very reason that he has not had the treatment you name; he has his blood and vital energies, unimpaired by the treatment, to sustain him. " And he did not die, but recovered, and was appointed Governor of one of the Western Territories long after that.

After having practiced medicine for fifteen years, except the months I was absent at Cleveland the last six years of the time, I was invited to fill the chair of Theory and Practice in the New York Homoeopathic Medical College. This invitation I accepted, and removed to New York and took up my residence there, and commenced practice again in a new field. About the year 1868 I invented a new process for refining petroleum by the aid of superheated steam, and spent eighteen months in developing the process at Binghamton, N. Y., and then returned to my practice in New York City. In the year 1873 I gave up the practice of medicine, and in connection with two gentlemen who were interested in selling oils, I commenced the refining of petroleum, manufacturing therefrom machinery and other oils; to which business I have devoted my attention ever since. I have attended chiefly to the manufacturing department and my partners to the selling.

I have been frequently asked: "Why did you quit the practice of medicine? Was not that a useful business? " Yes, it was; but I had come to feel that there were fields for greater usefulness—in fact, that it was vastly more important to teach people the laws of health and life, and to strive to lead them by precept and example to shun the causes of disease, than it was to cure them when they were sick— that prevention was better than cure. Consequently, when I saw before me a reasonably sure prospect of being able to make a good deal more money at the refining business than I could ever expect to make in the practice of medicine, I could but feel that, by the aid of a reasonable portion of the money thus made, I could perform a far greater use than I could by practicing medicine. This, then, was the reason for my giving up a good and useful profession and practice for my present business. What I have attempted to do for the benefit of suffering humanity since I gave up the practice of medicine, I will name in a future chapter.

CHAPTER II.

WHY EVERY PHYSICIAN SHOULD EXAMINE AND TEST HOMOEOPATHY.

I was born in the year 1815, and on the 26th of November, 1891, was 76 years of age. I have not practiced medicine as a business for many years, and I never expect to practice again. As to money, my present business gives me all I need, and money to spare for benevolent purposes. I do not expect, nor do I desire, to receive one cent, directly or indirectly, for the writing of this pamphlet, or for the money which I expect to spend for paper, printing, binding, and sending it, post paid, to every physician and clergyman in the United States and Canada whose name I can get. I do it because I believe and hope it will be a useful work and instrumental in doing good, and that many who are willing and waiting will find useful suggestions contained in its pages, and that through their instrumentality humanity may be benefited.

A few years after I became a convert to Homoeopathy I met in a railroad car a venerable professor from the college where I graduated. We were mutually pleased to see each other, and after our congratulations were over I remarked to him that, so far as the administration of remedies was concerned, I had departed somewhat from the "general principles" which he used to inculcate, and that I had become a Homoeopathist. The Professor looked up with astonishment and exclaimed most earnestly: "I am sorry to hear that! I am sorry to hear that! " He manifested not the slightest desire to know why I had made the change, but was ready to denounce and condemn. It would be useless to talk to such a man. Before one can see a new truth, however plain it may be, he must be willing to either examine the question carefully himself, or to heed the testimony of those who have examined it. Fortunately, all physicians have not been like the above Professor; for there have been thousands who were educated in and graduated from Allopathic schools, some of them gray-haired men, who, like myself, have carefully studied Homoeopathy and cautiously tested the remedies upon the sick, who have become converts to the new practice, and who have ever after relied upon its remedies in the treatment of the sick. No intelligent physician of any other school has ever carefully read the Homoeopathic works, and has to any considerable extent cautiously used the remedies in the treatment of severe cases of various diseases, without being able to see the vast superiority of the Homoeopathic over the Allopathic treatment of disease; and no one, without prejudice, and willing to see the truth, will ever do so without being convinced. Can a man, with eyes open, on a clear day, go out at noon time and declare that the sun does not shine? He may make such a declaration while shut up in a cellar or cavern, or if he never opens his eyes. As one who has patiently and diligently studied and practiced both systems, I say without the slightest hesitation that Homoeopathy, as a system of practice, is as superior to Allopathy as the direct light of the sun is to the reflected light of the moon; in fact, much of the allopathic practice of to-day is but a reflection of the homoeopathic light. What intelligent physician to-day bleeds, blisters, salivates, or vomits his patients, as students were taught to do by preceptors, professors, and books fifty years ago? And why is such treatment so frequently, to say the least, discarded now by Allopathic physicians? Is it not largely because the success which results from the Homoeopathic treatment of diseases, has convinced Allopathic physicians and their patients that such violent disease-creating measures and remedies are unnecessary?

Homoeopathy is strictly a scientific system of medicine. It is based upon a law of nature—"*Similia similibus curantur,*" or the law that remedies will cure symptoms and diseases similar to those which they will cause when taken by healthy persons. It is wonderful with what care, skill, and perseverance the new Materia Medica has been developed, mostly by intelligent physicians, commencing with Hahnemann, taking the different remedies in varying doses, and carefully and patiently watching the symptoms that follow, and writing them down day after day; and then, when similar symptoms occur in case of disease, giving the remedies and carefully watching and writing down the results. Allopathic physicians, as a rule, have not the slightest conception of the vast amount of patient and persevering labor in this direction which has been done by physicians as well educated as they are, and most of whom have graduated in the same schools, who have devoted their lives to this work. Are not these facts worthy of the consideration of every physician in the world who desires the highest good of his fellow men? It is well known to every intelligent physician that there is some truth in the homoeopathic law of cure, and that it has to some extent been recognized from the earliest periods of medical history. A cathartic remedy, even in Allopathic doses, will sometimes cure a diarrhoea, and an emetic will sometimes cure a nauseated stomach; but such remedies when given in large doses do not always cure, or they would generally be used by Allopathists; they sometimes seriously and even dangerously aggravate the disease, so that the vital forces do not react and thus effect a cure. Nitrate of silver and acetate of zinc, which applied to well eyes will cause irritation and inflammation, are often applied to inflamed eyes. The kine pox, which is a similar disease, is well known to either prevent or materially modify smallpox; and so I could go on enumerating cases where Allopathic physicians treat their patients in accordance with the Homoeopathic law of cure. The great discovery of Hahnemann was not so much the Homoeopathic law of cure, for some knowledge of that was possessed before his day, but the practical application of that law to the cure of disease. He found by careful experiments that diseases can be cured by remedies, which when given to the well will produce similar symptoms or diseases, in doses so small as not to seriously aggravate the existing disease or symptoms; and that all diseases may be thus treated with a success hitherto unknown. This discovery was accompanied by the most careful experiments by him and his followers upon themselves, to ascertain with the greatest possible care the effects of various remedies upon the healthy, so as to be able to make accurate prescriptions for the sick. Here you have most careful scientific investigation and experiments as to the action of remedies upon the well and sick, made, not by pretenders or quacks, but by well educated physicians, that should command the admiration and respect of every intelligent man and educated physician.

As to the doses given to the sick, which have been such a stumbling-block to our Allopathic brethren, their size is simply the result of the most careful experiments. Everyone can understand that if we give an Allopathic dose of Ipecac to a patient already sick and vomiting, or of Veratrum album to a patient suffering from Asiatic cholera or cholera morbus, we will almost certainly aggravate the disease, perhaps to a fatal extent; for it is the reaction of the vital forces of the system against the new excitement caused by the remedy, which overcomes this new excitement and the diseased action at the same time. Now, if the action of the remedy is so severe that no reaction follows, then, of course, no cure follows, and even death may result.

The great beauty and excellence of the Homoeopathic system of medicine consists in the ability to treat patients successfully thereby, without making well organs sick, or aggravating existing diseased action, or creating an opposite diseased state, as you do when you give a cathartic remedy in a cathartic dose for constipation; in that

Personal Experience of a Physician

case the reaction, if reaction follows, is not in the right direction, consequently the constipation is often aggravated. I have hardly ever seen, excepting in cases of mechanical obstruction, a severe and troublesome case of constipation that had not been caused by the use of cathartic remedies. So if we give an opiate, or an astringent, for a diarrhoea, we can see that it is a direct effort to restrain the disease by force, as it were, and we necessarily have to give large doses; and, if the vital forces react against this medicinal intrusion, the reaction is not in the direction of health. It is true that the vital forces sometimes overcome the diseased action in spite of the medicinal action; but it does not always do this, and subacute and chronic diarrhoeas are the result of the use of such remedies in some cases. To create disease of a well organ for the sake of curing disease in another organ, as is done when blisters are applied to the skin for diseases of internal organs, and when cathartics are given for diseases of the head or lungs, every one can see is a roundabout treatment; and while patients may sometimes be benefited by this calling off, as it were, the attention of the vital forces from the diseased action in other organs, still it is not a very satisfactory treatment as a whole; for you may lessen the vital power of resistance against diseased action, and may even cause serious disease of the organ assailed. I repeat, one of the great beauties of Homoeopathy lies in the fact that when remedies are given in accordance with its law of cure, they do not have to be given in disease-creating doses.

Hahnemann tells us that a single dose of the 30th dilution of Aconite, which contains but the decillionth of a drop of the tincture of the remedy, will cure acute pleurisy in twenty-four hours. I have thus treated patients suffering from pleurisy with a single dose of that remedy (it should be given soon after the commencement of the disease), and at the end of twenty-four hours have found the pain and fever all gone, and the skin moist and cool; and in one instance within two days the patient was on his way to California. I have never seen any such satisfactory cures of that disease from any kind of Allopathic treatment, nor from the low dilutions of Aconite or any other Homoeopathic remedy.

Hereafter I shall call attention of both physicians and the clergy to the causes and different methods of restraining or curing both spiritual and natural diseases; for there is the most beautiful analogy or correspondence between the methods of treating natural and spiritual diseases, and they must be considered in connection if we would clearly see the truth.

CHAPTER III.

THE DANGERS THAT RESULT FROM THE ALLOPATHIC TREATMENT OF DISEASES.

This treatment of diseases, more in the past than at present, consists largely in giving and applying remedies in disease-creating doses. The antiphlogistic treatment consists of blood-letting and the use and application of reducing remedies which directly or indirectly lessen the inflammatory or febrile action; but it is manifest that while it may lessen the activity of the diseased symptoms it also lessens the vitality of the system as a whole, and consequently its power to resist and overcome the existing diseased action; so that it is a serious question whether in many cases more is not lost than gained, and it is certain that, owing to the loss of blood and strength, convalescence will be more tedious. Then the use of remedies which cause active diseased action is not always safe. My own mother, at the age of 51 years, while in delicate health, was taken with a severe pain in her side. A physician was called. She thought an emetic would do her good. The physician gave her one, and she died during its operation, or immediately afterward. Her physician was so affected by this sudden and unexpected result that he had to go and lie down. At that time I was but 10 years old.

In typhoid fever there is a tendency to irritation of the mucous membrane of the small intestines; and, as I have already stated, I am satisfied from observation that when cathartics are given during this disease this irritation is often most seriously aggravated, and death not unfrequently follows as a result.

But the greatest danger and evil which result from the Allopathic treatment of disease lie, not in the direction of the sudden deaths which sometimes result from the use of its remedies, but in the liability of patients to be led into the habitual use of a drug that has afforded them palliative relief during sickness, and the countenance thus given for the use of such drugs by the laity during health. Perhaps as a rule poisonous substances palliate the symptoms which they cause, or which follow their use. A cathartic remedy will palliate the costiveness which frequently follows the use of cathartic remedies. Opium will palliate the sleeplessness and suffering that follow when the patient leaves off the use of opiates which he has been taking for disease; and alcohol and all fluids and remedies which contain an appreciable quantity of alcohol will palliate the coldness of the surface, craving, and distress which follow when a patient who has been taking such remedies attempts to discontinue their use. And thus the patient is led to continue the remedy because it makes him feel better every time he takes it; and, consequently, he is led on as naturally as water runs down hill, until he becomes a slave to his appetite.

Now, cannot every conscientious and intelligent man see what an immense blessing to his fellow men it would be if all physicians were able to treat their patients as successfully by the use of Homoeopathic remedies and doses as by the use of the so-called Alcoholic stimulants and Narcotics, which are enslaving and ruining so many, and thus be able to discard and discountenance the use of all such remedies? How can honest, conscientious physicians disregard and treat with contempt the testimony of physicians who have been educated in the same schools with themselves, but who have used their reason and freedom to investigate the new practice and test the curative action of its remedies, when they assure them that they have treated their patients far more successfully by the use of Homoeopathic remedies than they ever have done by the use of narcotics, alcoholic and fermented drinks, and other Allopathic remedies? How can physicians disregard the testimony of multitudes of patients who have been thus cured?

Why should not every physician study Homoeopathy and test the remedies on the sick? He can do it cautiously; he has all of his old remedies by him; what has he to lose? If they do not relieve his patient's sufferings more safely and promptly, he is not obliged to continue to use them. Is it a sensible and rational course for any one to allow himself to be so strongly confirmed in the views of prominent professors, teachers, and books, that he cannot without prejudice examine new truths and new methods of treating diseases, and even new theories? Should not a man strive to keep abreast of the age in which he is living? Take it, for instance, in regard to the action of alcohol on living structures. No other man has ever experimented so carefully, patiently, and thoroughly as has Dr. Richardson, of England, and the results of his experiments appeal to the common sense and observation of every unbiased man. He shows conclusively by its action that it should never have been given in a vast majority of the cases of disease where it is given by physicians; yet what attention is paid to his testimony and demonstrations, which every disinterested physician can see to be true if he will?

Dr. Richardson has also shown conclusively that alcohol paralyzes the minute capillary vessels, so that while the blood is forced into them through the arteries by the heart, it does not flow out of these minute vessels into the veins as rapidly as it does during their healthy action; consequently these vessels are congested and unnaturally distended with blood; the face and surface of the body become red, owing to the presence of an unnatural quantity of blood in these vessels. Nor is this all. The heat of the body is generated by changes going on in the blood and flows with the blood, and consequently the surface of the body becomes, from the presence of this excess of blood, unnaturally warm; but the heat is rapidly radiated from the surface, consequently the body, as a whole, becomes cooler. Dr. Richardson found by careful experiment that, while the surface was warmer, internally the body was cooler and less able to stand the cold; and he also substantiated the truth of his experiments by experiments on pigeons.

I will allow Canon Wilberforce, of South Hampton, England, to describe his experiment. While attending a reception during his recent visit to New York he was asked the following question: —

Dr. E. P. Thwing: "I would like to ask the Canon, as a physician, if the feeling as to alcoholic medication in England has changed for the better; for instance, the aspect of the British Medical Association toward this subject?"

Canon Wilberforce: "I believe that is one point in which we are going furthest ahead. I think that the whole aspect of the medical question is changing, mainly under the influence of that distinguished man of science, Dr. Richardson. He is one of the leading scientific minds of Great Britain. He has been successful in his experiments and as bold as a lion in his utterances, and he is leading scientific thought in this direction. He has proved over and over again, to use a common phrase, that from the monarch on the throne down to the maggot in the cheese, every healthy being is better without alcohol. The other day he was staying with me. I have the greatest possible objection to experimenting upon living animals, but he described to me an experiment on pigeons. It was not a very painful experiment; indeed, there are some people who, I am afraid, would like to have the experiment made upon them. He tried to induce the pigeons to take peas soaked in alcohol. They refused to do so at first; but after a while they were pleased, and they selected the peas saturated with alcohol. One cold night he turned the pigeons out, and on the following day, when he was examining them, strange to say, all those pigeons that ate the alcoholized peas were frozen to death, and those that remained teetotalers were perfectly safe and sound."

The drinking of alcoholic liquors generates no heat, it simply holds the heat in the congested blood-vessels upon the surface of the body, where it is wasted, and thus the temperature of the body as a whole is lowered.

The greatest mortality which results from the use of intoxicating drinks does not result from what is recognized as drunkenness, but from what is recognized as moderate but steady drinking. The drunkard after his sprees usually has seasons of abstinence, during which he has a chance to recuperate or regain strength and vigor, and consequently drunkards often live to an advanced age; but the steady drinker has no such seasons of rest, but his face, by its almost constantly congested appearance, shows the condition of his internal organs; for the effect of alcohol is to paralyze the minute capillary vessels throughout the body and fill them with blood, which produces redness upon the surface and a sensation of warmth. The separation of waste and worn-out materials and their removal is largely effected through these minute blood-vessels, and it is through them that nourishment reaches all the structures of the body; consequently, the almost constant state of congestion of these minute vessels, which results from regular, moderate drinking, interferes very seriously with this change or purification and renewal of all the structures of the body. As a result, while some drinkers die from drunkenness, many more die from apoplexy, paralysis, laryngitis and bronchitis, heart failure, fatty degeneration of the heart, diseases of the stomach and liver, Bright's disease of the kidneys, etc., and especially from an inability to either resist or withstand epidemic, contagious, or inflammatory diseases, or even mechanical injuries.

There are life insurance companies that give special privileges to total abstainers over moderate drinkers (they never insure drunkards). Such companies find that they can give a bonus of from 17 to 23 per cent. to total abstainers as compared with moderate drinkers.

Personal Experience of a Physician

I remember very well attending the family of a brewer. He was standing by when I advised his wife not to drink beer, for it was not good for her, as it would increase her debility and retard her recovery. With astonishment and great emphasis he exclaimed: "Tell me that beer is not good for her! " Striking his chest with his fist, he said: "Just look at me and see what beer has done for me! " He was born in Scotland, and manifestly inherited a good, strong constitution. I replied to him: "You are a large, strong man, but a little too fleshy; what beer has done for you time will tell better than I can. " A few months, perhaps a year or two, after that conversation, I was riding up a street which led toward his residence when I was called in a hurry into a saloon to see a man who was said to have fallen down "in a fit. " On reaching his side I found the above brewer dead upon the floor. Without much question he died of heart failure, from fatty degeneration caused by the steady use of beer. I never heard of his being intoxicated.

Dr. W. B. Carpenter, who stands at the very head of the physiologists of our century, says: —

"That the taking of alcoholic stimulants is in any way useful in keeping up the heat of the body, may now be considered as a myth altogether exploded. "

Again he says: —

"Now, it is the result of many observations that the introduction of alcohol specially deranges the vaso-motor system; this derangement showing itself alike in disturbance of the heart's action, and in relaxation of the capillary vessels, which become filled with blood, especially in the nervous system and in the skin. This causes one to feel that warmth and exhilaration which is the first effect of the introduction of these disturbing agencies, and which are appealed to as evidence that drink does us good. Well, what are the facts? The fresh glow is simply the result of relaxation of the capillary vessels of the skin, allowing a large quantity of blood to come to the surface, so as to give the feeling of superficial warmth. But if a larger amount of blood comes to the surface, it robs the parts within; and the feeling of genial warmth gives way to a general depression, especially when we are exposed to severe cold. The temporary exhilaration of the nervous system, too, is followed by a corresponding depression. Hence a person feels 'sick and sorry' the next morning after taking alcoholic stimulant. "

As to alcohol giving strength, it is well known that it supplies no substance to the tissues; therefore it meets no want, and consequently can give no strength. Every one can see that blood-vessels, when paralyzed and congested with blood by alcohol, cannot perform their function in the metamorphosis of the tissues of the body, or of conveying nourishment to them and removing worn-out, effete substances from them, as during health. If you would see the legitimate effects of alcohol, look at the permanently congested face of the steady drinker, or his "rum blossoms, " and remember that the capillary vessels of his brain and other internal organs are in a similar state, and then say if you think he has been strengthened by alcoholic drinks.

I remember very well when a young man, when a neighboring farmer was sick and unable to gather his hay, that the young men in the neighborhood set a day when they would meet and gather his hay for him. When, on the day set, we met in the field, and the neighboring young men noticed that my brother and myself had no bottle of cider brandy with us, they exclaimed with delight, "We will lay you out before noon. " A spirited contest with our scythes commenced in good earnest. But they did not lay us out; they were glad to seek and lie in the shade of trees to rest, while we were able to continue our work. It is well known that men who are preparing themselves for, or engaging in, feats requiring great strength and endurance are beginning to find that they must let intoxicating drinks alone. It is something marvelous to see with what tenacity so many physicians hold on to the idea that fermented wine, beer, brandy, and whiskey are strengthening. This idea comes, to a great extent, from the custom which prevails of giving such drinks to patients who are recovering from fevers, acute diseases, and from the effects of other debilitating causes. Many physicians have been so accustomed to give these drinks to patients, under such circumstances, that they have not the slightest idea how much better they would do without them.

A few years ago I met a German woman whose husband I knew well, and had reason to fear that beer drinking was doing him great harm. I said to her that, on her husband's account, she should never let another drop of beer enter her house if she could help it. "Why, " she exclaimed, "I cannot do without beer. I suffer so much during and after confinement, and am so weak, and have so little milk for my child, that my doctor says that I must have beer to give me strength. " She was then expecting to be confined within a few months. I replied to her by saying: "I have attended a great many more patients during confinement than your physician has ever attended, and after the first three years of my practice, I never gave to a single patient beer, fermented wine, whiskey, or brandy, or any other intoxicating drink. Now, if you will follow my advice, you will have a very different time from what you have ever had before; and my advice is that from this time forth you do not taste a single drop of beer, wine, or any other intoxicating drink. " She said she would follow my suggestions. I met her again when her child was a few months old, and she looked like another woman. She came up to me and said: "Well, Doctor, I have followed your advice strictly. I have not tasted beer, wine, or any other intoxicating drink, and I never before had such a comfortable time during my confinement. I never was so strong or gained my strength so rapidly. I never had so much nurse for my child, and I never had such a good-natured baby before. " She was the mother of several children.

Such are the results of the two methods of treatment.

There is no surer way to retard and often prevent recovery than to give patients drinks or even remedies which contain an appreciable quantity of alcohol. Where the tendency to recovery is strong they will recover sooner or later in spite of the treatment; but in some cases the physician may keep a delicate, nervous patient sick as long as he gives alcohol in any form; and in the most critical stage of typhoid fever, pneumonia, and other diseases where the patient needs nourishment, and that impurities should be removed, there is no more dangerous treatment than to give alcohol in any form, which interferes with these processes by paralyzing and congesting the capillary vessels. Hot water and nourishment, cautiously supplied, are what such patients require, not alcoholic stimulants.

The habit of taking either opium or morphine in our country has very generally resulted from the prescriptions of physicians. The patient may obtain palliative relief from its use, but suffers when he attempts to leave it off; consequently, without fully realizing the danger which he incurs, he continues the remedy until he is enslaved.

With the exception of alcohol, I know of no more dangerous medicine to give during the critical stages of inflammatory, febrile, and other diseases than Allopathic doses of opium in any form. This anodyne, by its retarding, benumbing, and stupefying effects upon the body, often destroys the power of reaction at the critical stage of the disease when the vital forces should be left free to act, and consequently in many cases patients die who would not die if they were not under the influence of this drug. Patients will often go very near to the border line and yet rally if kept free from the so-called "stimulants" and narcotics, and simple, plain nourishment is cautiously given and the body kept warm.

Physicians are sometimes responsible for the habit of using tobacco among their patrons. It is generally in chronic cases of disease where tobacco is prescribed, and, as a rule, when it is once prescribed by a physician the patient never thinks of giving up the use of the remedy; nor, so far as I have known, are physicians who prescribe tobacco often, if ever, careful to direct patients to discontinue using the remedy as soon as the symptoms of the disease from which they are suffering are relieved. Of course, a physician who neglects to do this seriously neglects his duty. It is safe to say that few physicians ever prescribe the smoking or chewing of tobacco as a remedy for diseases who do not use the weed themselves, for they can generally find much better and safer remedies.

If a physician loves intoxicating drinks and has become a slave to them, he actually feels that they do him good every time he drinks, for by relieving the symptoms temporarily which they have caused they actually make him feel better; and what is more natural than that he should prescribe them for his patients? Here, then, it can be clearly seen that there is great danger in employing physicians who love intoxicating drinks, tobacco, or opium in any form; for they believe in the efficacy of these poisons, and they will often prescribe them when a physician not addicted to their use would not think of doing so.

I have alluded to some of the dangers which attend and the evils which often result from the Allopathic treatment of diseases. Every one can see that they are formidable enough and that they merit the serious attention of every lover of his race. The skillful homoeopathic physician is able to avoid these dangers and evils, for he does not use disease-creating or appetite-begetting doses of any remedy.

We notice that those having the management of our railroads are beginning to see that, for the protection of the property of the owners and lives of their patrons, it is not safe to employ men who drink intoxicating drinks at all; for it is well known that large numbers of those who drink are sooner or later sure to become unreliable and careless. Is it not time that physicians should cease to accept as students, and that our medical colleges should cease to graduate and send forth as physicians, men who drink intoxicating drinks? Should not medical professors and teachers have as much regard for the health and lives of men, women, and children as the managers of our railroads?

Again, it is well known that the use of tobacco tends to prevent development, impair health, and to make men moody, if not careless, and it not unfrequently leads them, especially when young, to disregard the rights and feelings of others. We see men and boys smoking wherever it is not strictly prohibited, even lighting their cigars and cigarettes as they leave our elevated railroad stations, and walking down the stairs before ladies and gentlemen, thus compelling those who follow to breathe the atmosphere which they have polluted. As a fair illustration of the spirit so frequently manifested, I will describe a little incident which occurred in my presence. A young man, perhaps twenty years old, stood in a line of men approaching the paying teller's window in one of our banks, vigorously smoking his cigar. An elderly gentleman behind him asked him if he would be so kind as not to smoke. The young man immediately straightened himself up in a most self-important manner and exclaimed: "What do you think I care if it is offensive to you?"

In our railroad cars smokers have to separate themselves from wives, children, and friends and go by themselves into a smoking-car or apartment, and why? simply because tobacco smoke is unpleasant to every man, woman, and child who is not accustomed to it; and the smoker's breath often smells so strong of the smoke when his cigar is gone that it is exceedingly unpleasant to sensitive persons. Why should our medical colleges graduate young men to go forth for the purpose of attempting to heal sick, sensitive, and nervous patients, who smoke or chew tobacco, and thus are unpleasant to many and a bad example to all? Have we not enough cleanly young men, of good habits, to supply all the physicians we need in our country? A smoking physician, by his breath and bad example to the young, may do a vast deal more harm than he can ever do good as a physician in the world.

The use of an intoxicating wine as a communion wine in so many of our churches, and the efforts of so many clergymen to justify its use, together with the prescription of intoxicating drinks by physicians, are the chief supports which to-day sustain our distilleries, breweries, and saloons, and the prevalent drinking habits and consequent drunkenness. Let all of our clergy, churches, and physicians withdraw their patronage and sanction of intoxicating drinks, and it would not be many years before the manufacture and sale of such drinks would be prohibited throughout the length and breadth of our land. That day will surely come, for a new age is opening up before us very different from the past. The Lord is coming at this day in the "clouds of heaven" with power and great glory. Old things are passing away and all things are being made new—new heavens and a new earth.

Sir Astley Cooper says: "I never suffer ardent spirits in my house, thinking them evil spirits. If the poor could witness the white livers, the dropsies, or the shattered nervous systems which I have seen, the consequences of drinking, they would be aware that spirits and poisons are synonymous terms."

Again he says: "We have all been in error in recommending wine as a tonic. Ardent spirits and poisons are convertible terms."

Dr. Benj. Richardson declares it to be his opinion that the administration of alcohol will become, like blood-letting, a thing of the past, that it is passing into the same position as blood-letting. He, as a student, was educated to bleed; he was educated in the employment of alcohol; he saw the effects of the application of these tested by comparison, and he has, in one instance as much as in the other, come to consider them as behind the age, and both as remedies belonging to a departed and deceived generation. —The Dawn (English), Nov. 19, 1891.

I cannot close this chapter without again earnestly calling the attention of all physicians to the great danger to life which results from giving alcohol in any form to patients in very critical cases, or as they are at or approaching the crisis in their disease, in fevers and in inflammatory diseases, such as pneumonia, etc.

Since writing the preceding pages, in fact, since most of them were in type, my attention has been called by notices in our papers to the fact that champagne was given to a starving man, and that a few drops of brandy were mixed with the milk given to a child in a similar condition, or suffering from marasmus; and within a week a physician who has traveled extensively and lectured before medical, theological, and literary organizations, and who has frequently been in consultation in critical cases, described in my hearing several cases of pneumonia which he visited, which were, as he expressed it, drunk. When asked by the attending physician what he would suggest, he always replied, "Stop giving your patients alcoholic liquids; " and with a single exception, out of a large number, and that was a complicated case, recovery followed. While practicing in Detroit I was called to see a prominent citizen who was suffering from typhoid fever. His physicians had told his family that he would die, but that the "stimulants" they were giving him might keep him alive a few hours. I found him delirious, with cold, clammy extremities and almost pulseless. I stopped his "stimulants" at once and gave him Homoeopathic remedies and nourishment, and the next day he was out of danger. No more dangerous treatment has ever been adopted than to give a patient in a critical stage of disease alcohol in any form or quantity. Every intelligent physician ought to be able to see that this is true. I repeat, alcohol paralyzes the minute capillary vessels and veins (look at the face of the drinker) on the surface of the body, in the brain (look at a drinker's words and actions), stomach, lungs, and kidneys, and congests them with blood, through which the structures are nourished with food and drink and purified by the removal of decomposed and effete substances. Cannot every one see that these vessels, when thus paralyzed and congested, cannot perform their duty as well as they can in a natural state? Then, again, the temperature of the body is lowered internally and its heat wasted from the surface. What patients in the critical stages of disease require are warmth applied, if needed, to the surface of the body and limbs, and hot water (not scalding hot, of course), milk, unfermented wine, and other simple, easily digested articles which will nourish and strengthen the body taken internally.

It is possible that in sudden, severe cases of hemorrhage, alcohol may sometimes rescue a patient from fainting and bleeding to death, by storing the blood in the capillary vessels of the brain and surface of the body temporarily while the bleeding vessels contract; but even in such cases other remedies, if at hand, may prove more reliable.

In cases of marasmus in children, if Homoeopathic remedies and nourishing articles fail to give relief, and the child becomes greatly emaciated, give the child cautiously salt fat pork, fried, but not to a crisp; give him a piece in his hand, too large for him to swallow, and see with what avidity he will chew and suck it. The fat in combination with the salt will supply a want in the child's system, and patients will often be restored by this simple treatment after other measures have failed.

Even if alcohol were a stimulant, as some claim, we can certainly see that to give it to a patient in a state of great exhaustion, either from lack of nourishment or from an inability to take nourishment owing to diseased action, is to most seriously endanger the life of the patient and often to destroy life; for alcohol gives no nourishment, and all unnatural excitement is necessarily followed by corresponding depression, which often carries patients in critical cases below the living point, and death follows.

I will close with the following from the *Health Monthly*: —"The theory that whiskey is necessary in the treatment of pneumonia has received a blow from Dr. Bull, of New York, who discovers that in the New York hospitals sixty-five per cent. of the pneumonia patients die with alcoholic treatment, while in London, at the Object Lesson Temperance Hospital, only five per cent. die. —*Ex.*"

CHAPTER IV.

PERSONAL RELIGIOUS EXPERIENCE OF A PHYSICIAN; AND AN APPEAL IN BEHALF OF A NEW DISPENSATION.

We know that in various ages of the world the Lord has revealed a knowledge of Himself to man. In the Ten Commandments we have the laws of spiritual life, in accordance with which we must live if we would enjoy spiritual health, precisely as we must live in accordance with the laws of natural life and health, if we would enjoy natural health.

We are dependent upon revelation for a knowledge of the laws of spiritual health, and of the causes and methods for the cure of spiritual diseases; but the Lord gives us, if we will keep His sayings, the ability, by careful scientific study and investigation, to obtain a knowledge of the physical laws of health, and the causes and methods of curing physical diseases. And it is wonderful how the natural in all respects symbolizes or corresponds to the spiritual.

To the Jewish Church the Lord revealed so much knowledge of Himself, and how they should live if they would be prosperous and happy here and hereafter, as that Church was prepared to receive; and He also promised to manifest Himself in person. All Christians believe that He fulfilled His promise when Jesus Christ appeared on earth; but He did not come in the manner which the Jews at the time of His advent expected. He came, not as a temporal ruler or prince; consequently they took Him for an impostor and crucified Him. To His followers and disciples He promised to come again in the clouds of heaven; but the clouds of heaven may not be the clouds of the material earth, any more than the spiritual kingdom which He came to establish was a natural kingdom; and it is possible that His second coming may not be in the manner anticipated by the Christian Church at the time of His second coming. He intimated as much when He inquired if He should find faith on earth. Should Christians, then, not watch and pray, and heed the signs of the times, lest they follow the example of the Jews, and reject Him at His second coming? Should not clergymen, as well as physicians, be led in freedom according to reason, and not blindly by prominent religious professors, clergymen and writers, and creeds formulated in an age of comparative darkness? Should the traditions and creeds of men be allowed to make of none effect the Word of God? Do we not see all around us signs of a most wonderful change going on in the world? Are these changes which we behold from the Lord, or from man?

I was reared in the Baptist Church. My father was a deacon, and labored faithfully to bring his children into the Church. I was taught that I must be converted, or get religion, before being baptized or joining the Church. What was meant by being converted I never fully comprehended, but I inferred from the instruction I received that it meant a radical change in one's feelings, the result of faith in the Lord's "atoning blood; " and that when this change was effected, I should be able to tell an experience similar to what I had heard others tell before joining the Church, which sometimes seemed quite marvelous. I attended "protracted meetings" and "revival meetings. " And, one evening, I remember hoping and almost feeling that I felt a little change, and I even thought of announcing my feelings in the meeting; but caution prevailed, and I concluded to wait until the next day and see if there really was any change in my feelings. When the next day came, I could see no change, and consequently I made no announcement. Thus, I grew up and continued, until I was over thirty years of age, outside of the organized Church. I always respected religion, the Bible, and religious teachers, but I never got converted.

I had many things during childhood and early youth to be thankful for. My father and grandfather before him were accustomed to gather the family, night and morning, and read, or have some member of the family read, a chapter in the Bible, and then prayer was offered. Now, when this is done regularly, and especially if the Bible is read, in course, with here and there a few kindly remarks by the father or mother, no one can tell the good impression which is made on the children; they learn to reverence the Bible, and, what is of exceeding great moment, they hear it read through and through several times before they reach manhood, and they become comparatively familiar with the good and living precepts therein contained. The Sabbath-school, once a week for an hour or two, is all very well; but, in my estimation, it is very little, compared with daily family worship and acknowledging the Lord, and asking a blessing. O, that all Christian men and women could be aroused to the importance of such religious observances?

Some years ago, I went with my wife and a friend for a summer outing to the Catskill Mountains, and spent a few days at the

Personal Experience of a Physician

Mountain House. There were a large number of guests there, of the various religious denominations. Those religiously inclined had established the custom of meeting every morning around a table, in a large room, when a chapter from the Bible was read, followed by singing and prayer. There have been few, if any, incidents of my whole life that I have more frequently thought of, or with greater pleasure and delight, than of those large, non-sectarian, and, as it were, family gatherings and simple services.

My mother died, as stated in the first part of this work, when I was ten years old. After remaining a widower for three years, during which period my grandparents, who lived with us, died and my only sister was married, my father married a widow, the mother of several children, a good Christian woman and a member of the Baptist Church.

I have always been thankful that I had a step-mother. No own mother could have been more kind, or have exercised a stronger influence for good over a son than she strove to exercise over me. She entered our home when I was thirteen years of age, when I needed a mother's influence and care perhaps as much as at any period of my life after I had ceased to draw my nourishment from my mother's breasts. Tears come into my eyes as I recall the pleasant, useful, and happy evenings and Sunday afternoons which I spent with her, when we happened to be alone in the house, reading and conversing about the interesting stories in the Bible and other religious books and papers that she thought would interest me. She may have had faults, yet I was about to say I do not remember one; but, unfortunately, she had one—she was a smoker of tobacco. Years before she had been troubled with "water brash, " and a physician who, without much question, was himself a smoker, advised her to smoke; so she commenced smoking. He did not tell her to stop smoking as soon as she felt relief, as any intelligent physician should have done, if he was so unwise as to make such a prescription; but it is a question whether she ever experienced any permanent relief; for she was a bright, intelligent woman, and would have been likely to stop smoking of her own accord if she had been cured. In my estimation the physician who made the prescription was much more to be blamed than she was for the habit which followed. But seventy years ago very little was known as to the fearful slavery and diseases and mortality which result from the use of tobacco, compared with what is known to-day. The sin of ignorance cannot be pleaded in extenuation of such habits to-day, as it could then.

Personal Experience of a Physician

As to intoxicating drinks, I remember hearing my grandfather, when he was over eighty years old, after taking a drink of cider-brandy, exclaim: "A good gift of God, if taken with faith and prayer."

Fortunately, or providentially, I would say, the temperance reformation commenced soon after, and my father and other prominent members and the clergymen of the Baptist and Congregational churches in our town took an active part in the new movement. My father signed the pledge not to drink intoxicating drinks, and I followed his example; and I thank the Lord that I did so, for it gave me the strength and courage to say, "No, I thank you, I never drink, " when invited and tempted to drink intoxicating drinks. No intoxicating drinks have been publicly sold in that town (Ashfield, Mass.) for many years. During a recent visit there I found that, within the past three years, there have been 61 deaths in the town, of whom 15 only were under 50 years of age, whereas 20 were over 80 years, of whom 4 were over 90 years of age. What do you think of that, Christian brother?

I remember very well the first ideas I had of God when a boy, which I derived from the preaching and praying of ministers. It was that God and our Lord Jesus Christ were two distinct Beings. We had for a time a venerable gray-headed old man who preached one Sabbath, and a young man who preached the next. I thought the old man represented God the Father and the young man represented Jesus Christ.

When I arrived at manhood and came in contact with men of different religious views, and read some of their writings, the doctrine of the Trinity became more and more a mystery to me. At one time I was slightly inclined to Unitarianism, but I could not reconcile their doctrines with the Bible. Yet the Trinitarians seemed to teach distinctly that there are either two Gods, possessing different attributes, or that Jesus Christ was not God. It does not make any difference what we say with our lips; the question is, What do we "think in our hearts"? When I heard a bishop of one of the prevailing denominations stand up in his pulpit, as I have, and represent Jesus Christ as standing with one hand upon the throne of Jehovah, and the other hand resting upon the sinner's head, pleading with the Father to forgive him for his (Christ's) sake, was there not in the mind of that bishop a distinct idea of two Beings, possessing different feelings and passions? Now, were both of them Gods, or was one of them not God? And when I heard prayers so frequently terminated by the phrase, "Forgive us for Christ's sake, " the question naturally arose, to whom were such prayers addressed? If there are any intelligent rational ideas connected with the phrase in the mind of the one using it, has not his prayer unquestionably been addressed to some God outside of the Lord Jesus Christ? Who is that God? Can Christian men safely reject the express teaching of our Lord Himself when on earth, when He declared: "I and my Father are One; " "Whose hath seen me, hath seen the Father"? and the apostle's teaching, that "God was in Christ, reconciling the world unto Himself"? Is there any other way to the Father at this day except through the person of the Lord Jesus Christ—God manifest in the flesh? Is He not the "Alpha and Omega, the beginning and the end, the first and the last"? Why, then, pray to an unknown God? In the Old Testament, we are told that "I, Jehovah, am your Savior, and beside me there is no Savior, " and in the New Testament we are told that in Jesus Christ dwelt all the fullness of the Godhead bodily. He is "Immanuel—God with us. " Let us, then, worship Him—One God in One Divine Person.

The doctrine of election and predestination early troubled me. I could not reconcile it with the loving kindness which the Sacred Scriptures proclaim as characteristic of our Heavenly Father.

The doctrine of justification by faith alone, "without the deeds of the law, " as the old hymn read, was not a doctrine which appealed to my reason, but it was a very consoling doctrine. Every young man who has been carefully reared by religious parents, and under the influences of a church, expects to be converted and get religion some time before he dies, and to join a church. But if he enjoys good health and the prospect of living for many years, especially if he is taught that, by merely believing or having faith at any time in the "atoning blood of Christ, " he can escape the consequences of his evil deeds, there is great danger of procrastination.

A clergyman once said to me: "If a man repents and gets converted one hour before his death, the worse he has been or lived, the happier he will be. " It seems to me better to be guided by the Word of the Lord, and to believe that the evil doer shall not go unpunished. The Lord came into the world to save men from sin and from the penalty only so far as they co-operate with Him. Sin is the cause, the penalty is the effect; and effect follows cause as a normal and necessary consequence.

Personal Experience of a Physician

The young, as well as the old, should be taught the great truth, that every thought we harbor, and every word we speak, and every act we do, aid in building up our spiritual organism, and will tell on our eternal destiny, just as the natural food and drink we use, and the exercise we take, will tell on the future health of our material bodies, for good or evil; and there is no avoiding it. If a man or woman, young or old, would be right in the future, he must do right in the present. No one should forget that, even if we reach heaven, the mansion which we will occupy there will depend on our lives here—every one will unite with those like Himself. No one can tell the immense harm which has been done to our race, by teaching that either by faith alone, or through the influence or efforts of the clergy, men can be saved from the penalties or consequences which are sure to follow an evil life. The "willing and obedient" shall eat the good of the land. Our blessed Lord tells us: "If ye keep my commandments, ye shall abide in my love" (John xv: 10). Thus beautiful, symmetrical, spiritual organisms are built up, not by "sowing wild oats" during youth, and disobeying the divine commandments during the subsequent period of life. It is well for all, young or old, to remember the Word: "Be not deceived; God is not mocked: for whatsoever a man soweth, that shall he also reap. " (Gal. vi: 7.) At this day we need practical doctrines, which shall unite religion and life, or faith and charity, and such alone will command the respect of non-churchgoers.

While a young man my attention was early called to the doctrines of the Universalists, but their doctrines did not seem to me to accord with the Sacred Scriptures; nor did I think that all men could be equally happy hereafter, when there is such a vast difference in their conduct and lives here. Genuine happiness is the result of right willing and doing; in other words, of keeping the commandments. I have no doubt but the Lord desires that all men should thus live and be happy; but we know that all men are not willing. Having created them free agents, God does not compel them here to love the Lord and their neighbor, which loves manifestly constitute heaven; what reason, then, have we to think He will compel them to do it hereafter? If a man deliberately leads an evil life here, growing ever stronger and more confirmed in that life, until he has made evil his good and rejoices in it, what reason have we to suppose or assume that he will change when he enters the next life? I am willing to leave him in the hands of the Lord—he has passed from my sight. I well remember the remarks of my grandmother when she was eighty-six years of age, a few days after the death of her husband, my grandfather. She said: "I do not fear to die, for I feel that God will do me no injustice. " Within a few days she departed in peace.

The Millerite excitement commenced when I was a young man. When I was about twenty years old I was traveling in central Massachusetts. One night there was a meeting of Millerites in the neighborhood where I was stopping, and I attended the meeting. The speaker was very zealous and earnest in his remarks. There was a comet with quite a long tail then visible, and he seemed to think that that comet, with its tail, might sweep across the track of our earth and work its destruction, which he anticipated. I remember very well my reflections on leaving that meeting. A few days before I had stood upon the side of a hill near the track, and had seen for the first time a railroad train on its way from Boston to Worcester. I said to myself: "Now we have railroads, steamboats, friction matches, temperance societies, Sunday-schools, the Bible translated into various languages, which but a few years ago were unknown. This great continent, from being a wilderness, inhabited by a comparatively few wild Indians, has been discovered and is being developed and cultivated by civilized and Christian people, and gradually being made capable of containing and sustaining hundreds of millions of inhabitants. " With all these facts before me, I said to myself, "It looks a great deal more as though the world is just beginning to live; in fact, that a new era is dawning, than it does that the world is going to be destroyed. " From that night the Millerite doctrine never troubled me any more, for I felt that I beheld, in all the wonderful inventions being made and changes going on in the world, the dawning light of a better day for the inhabitants of our earth.

CHAPTER V.

THE DAWN OF A NEW DISPENSATION.

We behold the dawn of a new day before we see the sun, from whence the light proceeds.

The young in the Baptist Church, not having been baptized in infancy, are brought up to feel that they are out of the Church, and that they have to be converted, or "to get religion, " before they join the Church, instead of being brought up to feel that, having been baptized, they belong to the Church and must believe its doctrines, and live the life which they teach. Thus I remained out of the Church until I was over thirty years of age. After I was twenty-three years old I attended different churches, as was most convenient. For a time I attended the Episcopal Church, while studying medicine; and after I graduated I attended the Congregational Church for several years more frequently than any other; but I had no thought of joining that Church, for during those days I always thought that immersion was the only true mode of baptism.

While practicing medicine in Detroit, a gentleman whose family I was attending asked me if I would not like to read a work on "Heaven and Hell, " written by Emanuel Swedenborg, who claimed, he said, to have had open intercourse with the spiritual world, and to have written of what he had seen and heard in that world. He said that he had read it, and believed that the views therein contained were rational and true. If I had ever heard of them at all, at that time, I had never heard the writings of Swendenborg spoken of favorably before. Out of respect to the gentleman, I took the book home with me, but did not feel sufficient interest in it to attempt to read it through in course, but read here and there a few pages; and, after keeping it a few weeks, I returned it to the owner, feeling from what I had read no interest in its contents. Not long after this a lady whom I was attending asked me if I would not like to read Professor George Bush's reasons for accepting as true the revelations contained in the writings of Emanuel Swedenborg. Well, I thought to myself, if the gentleman who lent me "Heaven and Hell, " if my patient here, who is a very intelligent woman, and Professor Bush, whom I had understood was a very learned man, believe that Swedenborg's writings contain truths good and useful, it may be well for me to read the pamphlet then before me. So I took the book home with me and commenced reading it. About that time Rev. George Field commenced the delivery of a course of lectures on Creation and the first chapters of Genesis, treating the subject from the standpoint of Swedenborg's writings. I attended his lectures, which added very much to my interest, and I read Bush's reasons with care. Then I obtained "Heaven and Hell, " and read it carefully through with the greatest interest. When a small boy I remember very well listening with fear and trembling to a discourse delivered by a clergyman, on "God is angry with the wicked every day, " in which the speaker dwelt upon the fearful sufferings which the Lord had in reserve for the wicked in a hell of fire and brimstone, where they were to be tortured forever and ever.

When I came to read Swedenborg's "Heaven and Hell, " I found a very different and more rational doctrine taught—that heaven consists in loving the Lord and the neighbor, or in religious obedience to the divine commandments; and that hell consists in loving one's self and the world supremely, or sensual and selfish gratification, without regard to use; that either heaven or hell is within us, according to the character of our ruling love; that the Lord casts no one into hell, but does all He can, without interfering with man's freedom, to prevent men from going to hell; if they go there, they go of their own free choice, among their like, where selfishness in some form rules the hearts of the inhabitants; they would not and could not be happy among those who are ruled by love to the Lord and the neighbor; or by obedience to the divine commandments. The spiritual world is a more real world than this; therefore, in that world the motives, thoughts, and intentions of men cannot be hidden as readily as in this world; consequently, there is a great gulf between heaven and hell. One is opposite to the other. When love to the Lord and to the neighbor rules in the hearts of all the inhabitants, there is no need of penal laws or punishments, for each one is a law unto himself, and all are striving to do good to each other and to all; consequently, unity, peace, and harmony prevail.

How different from this is hell, where selfishness prevails; where the love of dominion over others, or the love of vain show, the love of acquiring unfairly that which belongs to others, the love of riches for the sake of being rich, and of selfish and sensual gratification without regard to use, rules in the hearts of all the inhabitants. We know that such perverted passions make a hell hot enough here; and, as death does not change the character of a man's ruling love, they will make a hell hot enough hereafter. But the Lord, in His mercy which endureth forever, by His angels governs the hells as well as the heavens, and does not permit vindictive punishments. All punishments are for the benefit of evil doers, to restrain and prevent them from doing evil to others and themselves, and from sinking to greater depths of wickedness; we may, therefore, safely leave the inhabitants of that world in His care.

No man or woman can read "Heaven and Hell" attentively, carefully, and prayerfully without great benefit. It is clearly shown that, to escape hell, an evil man has but to repent, to look to the Lord and shun evils as sins against Him, and that the Lord is no respecter of persons, but that He gives to every man the ability to do this, if he is willing. When we examine ourselves carefully in the light of the Sacred Scriptures, and discover an evil, if we shun that evil as a sin against the Lord, He keeps us in the effort to shun all evils, and enables us more clearly to see other evils to which we are inclined. Here is an open door for approaching the Lord, free to all; there is no mystery about it. If an evil man is to be reformed, he must repent or face about and commence a life of shunning evils as sins against God; otherwise, there will be no radical change, but a miserable shuffling from one evil habit to another. Even if a man shuns one evil habit, like the smoking or chewing of tobacco, because it injures his health and is likely to destroy his life, and not because it is a sin, and without the acknowledgment that it is a sin, he is almost sure to seek as a substitute some form of intoxicating drinks—opium, strong coffee, or tea. We make a great mistake, as Christians, if we try to substitute coffee- or tea-houses for saloons; not that the effects of coffee and tea are as pernicious as intoxicants, but they are unnecessary, and often diseases and great suffering result from their use. We should strive to show men and women, in the light of this day, what substances are unmistakably injurious to health and endanger life, and strive to lead them, by precept and example, to shun their use as sins against God.

After reading "Heaven and Hell" I read the "True Christian Religion, " which is the last work that Swedenborg published, containing the essential doctrines of the New Christian Church, or the New Jerusalem now descending from God out of Heaven, "making all things new. " In this work it is clearly shown that God is one in essence and in person, and that in the Lord Jesus Christ that one God is manifested to men. God is love. "In the beginning was the Word and the Word was, with God and the Word was God. " Here we have the Father or Divine Love, the Son or Divine Wisdom, and the

Holy Spirit or Divine Proceeding, flowing from the Father because He is a being of infinite love, wisdom, and power, through the Son, a trinity in unity. The Divine Being is no more three persons than a man is three persons, because he is created in the image of God and has affection or love, an understanding, or thoughts, words, and acts that flow from his love through his understanding out toward his fellow men. All the doctrines of the New Christianity are based upon the Sacred Scriptures and appeal to our highest reason; and we are to receive them because we see them to be true and in strict harmony with the Word when the latter is correctly understood.

But I have neither time nor space to discuss these doctrines here. I will simply say, that when we come to see clearly that there is but one God whose name is one, who was manifested in the person of the Lord Jesus Christ, and that whoso seeth Him seeth the Father, then a number of false doctrines which proceed from and cohere with the doctrine of a tri-personal Deity will disappear like mists before the rising sun; and we shall be prepared to see and understand the rest of the beautiful and rational doctrines taught in "The True Christian Religion, " and the mystery of Babylon and all man-made creeds will disappear before this new revelation from our Lord Jesus Christ.

After reading the "True Christian Religion" I read the work on Divine Providence, which gives such a clear view of the Lord's providential care over men that it strengthens and encourages the earnest seeker after truth wonderfully. It is a book which should be read by every Christian man and woman.

Next, "The Angelic Wisdom Concerning the Divine Love and Wisdom" throws a flood of light on the origin of the material universe and all created things. In this work we are clearly shown that the Lord is Love itself, because He is Life itself: and "that angels and men are recipients of life; " and "that all created things in a certain image represent man, " and "that Love is the life of man. "

But Swedenborg's "Apocalypse Revealed" was one of the most satisfactory works I ever read. It opened up to me a new world of thought, of expectation, hope and joy. The reading of this work and the first volume of his "Arcana Celestia" satisfied me that the Sacred Scriptures are divine or a special revelation from God to man, and differ from all merely human writings as much as a living man differs from a statue; for they are filled with a Divine spirit. The Lord says: "My words are spirit and life."

The Sacred Scriptures are written in accordance with the law of correspondence between spiritual and natural things. The spiritual is the cause, the natural is the effect; and effects must correspond to their causes in every particular. The Lord is the sun of the spiritual world and the creator of all things: consequently our natural sun corresponds to the spiritual sun, or the Lord. From the Lord, or the spiritual sun, love and wisdom proceed, and give life to man's spiritual body; from the natural sun flow natural heat and light which enable the natural body to live; natural heat and light therefore correspond to spiritual heat and light, or to love and truth, which are heat and light to the spirit of man. Through the natural clouds and atmosphere which surround the earth we receive natural heat and light from the natural sun, as we receive spiritual heat and light or love and truth from the Lord through the literal sense of the Sacred Scriptures; Consequently the clouds of heaven in which the Lord was to come are the literal sense of his holy Word, unfolding its spirit and life and manifesting the Father clearly to His children. The sun which was to be darkened was not the natural but the spiritual sun, or the Lord obscured to man's spiritual perception. When men in their creeds separated the Lord into three persons, and framed doctrines in accordance therewith, which, in their estimation, would enable them to reach heaven by believing certain dogmas, instead of by a life according to the Divine Commandments, then was the sun indeed darkened in the minds of men. Then a true faith or knowledge of the Lord was destroyed and the moon became as blood. A true faith reflects the light or wisdom of the Lord upon man, as the natural moon reflects the light of the natural sun. Water corresponds to truth upon the natural plane of the mind, for it cleanses the natural body as truth cleanses his spirit; it also circulates throughout the natural body, conveying nourishment to all the structures of the body as truth circulates through the spiritual body, conveying that which is good and true to strengthen and develop the spiritual body. It is owing to this correspondence that water is used in the ordinance of baptism, for it performs the same office for the natural body that truth does for the spiritual body; it cleanses and conveys nourishment; and therefore baptism by water signifies that man is to be regenerated by receiving and living according to the truth. It is also the Christian sign—a sign that one baptized is of the Christian Church, or professes the Christian religion.

Personal Experience of a Physician

The "Fruit of the Vine, " or pure unfermented or unleavened wine, has been organized by the Lord in the vegetable kingdom; it therefore not only contains water, but also organized nourishment for the structures of the body, which supply in a most remarkable degree the wants of the body, like a mother's milk to her infant child; it therefore most beautifully symbolizes blood, and corresponds to spiritual truth, united with good from the Lord, which nourishes and builds up the spirit of man, when he drinks or appropriates it, or when he lives as divine truth teaches, shunning evils as sins against God. It is consequently used appropriately in the Most Holy Supper.

It has been my aim above to simply give the reader a glimpse of this most wonderful and beautiful of all sciences, and really the foundation of all sciences-the science of correspondence between natural and spiritual things. He who reads carefully and without prejudice the "Apocalypse Revealed" and the "Arcana Celestia, " with a desire to know and live according to the truth, cannot fail to see that the Sacred Scriptures are plenarily inspired, and are a special revelation from God to man; and that, different from all merely human writings, they contain within the letter a connected spiritual sense. That the science of correspondences was once understood by the inhabitants of our earth, is to be seen in the relics which remain in a more or less perverted form in the hieroglyphics of Egypt, the idolatry among many nations, and sun-worship, where the spiritual signification has often been lost and men have come to worship the natural objects instead of the spiritual, which they represent. The mythological writings of many nations, and even Masonry, contain remains of this once well known science. The first chapters of Genesis and the entire Word are written in strict accordance with this science. The first chapters of Genesis, like the Parables of our Lord, were not intended to be understood literally; the very names therein show this clearly. A tree of life, a tree of knowledge of good and evil, a talking serpent, how can any man for a moment suppose these to be natural trees and a natural snake? Do serpents ever talk? the garden eastward in Eden, and an Ark which would not hold the hides and teeth of all the animals on earth—were these to be understood literally?

CHAPTER VI.

A NEW DAY TO OUR EARTH.

"'Behold He cometh with clouds, ' signifies that the Lord will reveal Himself in the literal sense of the Word, and will open its spiritual sense at the end of the church. "—*A. R. 23.*

A church, we are taught, comes to its end when the true doctrines of the Word are falsified by its members, to justify evils of life; or when the members of a church who are in the love of ruling over others in civil and ecclesiastical affairs, for their own aggrandizement, or for vain show, or who love money or sensual gratification without regard to use, strive to justify the gratification of their perverted loves and appetites by an appeal to the Sacred Scriptures, and thus frame creeds and doctrines which exalt faith and ceremonials above a life of charity, and when men come to live in accordance with such false doctrines the church comes to its end. At the same time, there remain some who are still in the good of life, or striving to live good lives in obedience to the Divine commandments. Such comprise the common people who receive the Lord with joy at His coming, and follow Him, among whom a New Dispensation of Divine Truth commences. Such may be found both among the clergy and laity. The end of the world is the end of the Dispensation or Age, and not of the material earth—"The earth endureth forever. "

We are told by Swedenborg that the angels rejoiced greatly that it had pleased the Lord to reveal a knowledge of correspondences so deeply concealed during some thousands of years; "and they said it was done in order that the Christian Church which is founded on the Word, and is now at its end, may again revive and draw breath through heaven from the Lord. "—*Conjugial Love*, 532.

So we are not to look for the destruction of the prevailing religious organizations, but for the rejection of their false and irrational doctrines, and the receiving of new light and life from the Lord. And how is such a result to be brought about?

It was apparently the opinion of Swedenborg that his writings would be read by the clergy, who would teach the doctrines therein contained to their congregations; and thus the glorious truths for this new Era or crowning Church would be spread among the people;

for, in speaking of the descent of the New Church, or New Jerusalem, from God out of Heaven, he says it can only take place "in proportion as the falses of the former Church are removed; for what is new cannot gain admission where falses have before been implanted, unless those falses are first rooted out; and this must first take place among the clergy, and by their means among the laity."

That Swedenborg's anticipations are surely and somewhat rapidly being realized at this time seems beyond question; for over 30,000 clergymen of the various religious denominations of our country have already sent for and obtained Swedenborg's "True Christian Religion" and "Heaven and Hell," and over 25,000 have received his "Apocalypse Revealed." It is known that large numbers are reading the above works with great interest, and that hundreds if not thousands are full receivers of the doctrines therein contained, and that they are teaching them to their people as fast as they find they can receive them. In fact, many of Swedenborg's writings were translated into English by the late Rev. John Clowes, Rector of St. John's Church, Manchester, England, who, for many years, without ever being required to sever his connection with the Church of England, openly and boldly taught the doctrines revealed through Swedenborg. Mr. Clowes says: —

"Nothing, therefore, can be plainer than that the New Jerusalem Dispensation is to be universal, and to extend unto all people, nations, and languages on the face of the earth, to be a blessing unto such as are meet to receive a blessing. Sects and sectarians, as such, can find no place in this General Assembly of the ransomed of the Lord. All the little distinctions of modes, forms, and particular expressions of devotion and worship will be swallowed up and lost in the unlimited effusions of heavenly love, charity, and benevolence with which the hearts of every member of this glorious New Church and Body of Jesus Christ will overflow one toward another. Men will no longer judge one another as to the mere externals of church communion, be they perfect or imperfect; for they will be taught that whosoever acknowledges the incarnate Jehovah in heart and life, departing from evil, and doing what is right and good according to the commandments, he is a member of the New Jerusalem, a living stone in the Lord's new Temple, and a part of that great family in heaven and earth whose common Father and Head is Jesus Christ. Every one, therefore, will call his neighbor *Brother*, in whom he observes this spirit of pure charity; and he will ask no questions concerning the form of words which compose his creed, but will be satisfied with observing in him the purity and power of a heavenly life."

"The Gentiles," says Swedenborg, "cannot profane the holy things of the Church like Christians, because they are not acquainted with them." "They are afraid of Christians on account of their lives." "Those who have lived well, according to their religious principles, are instructed by the angels, and easily receive the truths of faith, and acknowledge the Lord," "for they have not formed for themselves any principles of falsity opposed to the truths of faith, which would need to be first removed."

"Although Gentiles are not in genuine truths during their life in the world, they receive them in the other life from a principle of love."

"The Church of the Lord exists with all in the universe who live in good according to their religious principles, and acknowledge the Divine Being; and they are accepted of the Lord and go to heaven."

The above is in strict accordance with all that Swedenborg has written; for he says: —

"In the spiritual world to which every man goes after death, it is not the character of your faith into which inquiry is made, nor of your *doctrine,* but of your *life,* whether it has been of this character or that; for it is known that such as a man's *life* is, such is his faith—nay, more, such is his doctrine; for life forms its doctrine and faith for itself." (D. P. 101.) "For the good of life according to one's religion contains within it the affection of knowing truths, which such persons also learn and receive when they come into the other life." (A. C. 455.)

"Evils which belong to the will, are what condemn a man and sink him down to hell; and falsities only so far as they become conjoined with evils; then one follows the other. This is proved by numerous instances of persons who are in falsities, and yet are saved." (*Ibid.* 845.)

"It has been provided that every one, in whatever heresy he may be as to the understanding, can still be reformed and saved, provided he shuns evils as sins, and does not confirm heretical falsities in himself; for by shunning evils as sins the will is reformed, and through the will the understanding, which then first comes out of darkness into light. There are three essentials of the Church: the acknowledgment of the Divine of the Lord, the acknowledgment of the holiness of the Word, and the life which is called charity. According to the life, which is charity, every one has faith; from the Word is the knowledge of what the life must be; and from the Lord are reformation and salvation. If the Church had held these three as essentials, intellectual dissensions would not have divided but only varied it, as light varies its colors in beautiful objects, and as various diadems give beauty in the crown of a king. " (*D. P.* 259.)

Here, then, we have a broad spirit of charity which acknowledges every man as a brother who believes in a Supreme Being, shuns evils as sins, and strives to live conscientiously and honestly according to the light he possesses.

As many who will be likely to receive this pamphlet may know little, if anything, in regard to the claims which Swedenborg makes, that he was the human instrument chosen by The Lord through whom to reveal to the world the truths of a New Dispensation, even of the Second Coming of the Son of Man, it may be well to allow this chosen servant to speak for himself as to his mission. He says: —

"I have been called to a holy office by the Lord Himself. I can sacredly and solemnly declare that the Lord Himself has been seen of me, and that He has sent me to do what I do, and for such purpose has opened and enlightened the interior part of my soul, which is my spirit, so that I can see what is in the spiritual world and those that are therein; and this privilege has now been continued to me for twenty-two years. But in the present state of infidelity, can the most solemn oath make such a thing credible or to be believed? Yet such as have received true Christian light and understanding will be convinced of the truths contained in my writings, which are particularly evident in the book of 'Revelations Revealed. ' Who, indeed, has hitherto known anything of importance of the spiritual sense of the Word of God, of the spiritual world, or of heaven and hell; the nature of the life of man, and the state of souls after the decease of the body? Is it to be supposed that these, and other things of like consequence, are to be eternally hidden from Christians? "

Again, in the "True Christian Religion, " at a later date, toward the close of his life in this world, he says: —

"I foresee that many who read the relations after the chapters, will believe that they are inventions of the imagination; but I assert in truth that they are not inventions, but were truly seen and heard; not seen and heard in any state of mind buried in sleep, but in a state of full wakefulness. For it has pleased the Lord to manifest Himself to me, and to send me to teach those things which will be of His New Church, which is meant by the New Jerusalem in the Revelation; for which end He has opened the interiors of my mind or spirit, by which it has been given me to be in the spiritual world with angels, and at the same time in the natural world with men, and this now for twenty-seven years."

In a letter to the King of Sweden, with characteristic simplicity and boldness, he says: —

"When my writings are read with attention and cool reflection (in which many things are to be met with hitherto unknown) it is easy enough to conclude that I could not come to such knowledge but by a real vision and converse with those who are in the spiritual world. I am ready to testify with the most solemn oath that can be offered in this matter, that I have said nothing but essential and real truth, without any admixture of deception. This knowledge is given to me by our Saviour, not for any particular merit of mine, but for the great concern of all Christians' salvation."

When asked why a philosopher was chosen to this office he replied: —

"To the end that the spiritual knowledge which is revealed at this day might be reasonably learned and naturally understood; because spiritual truths answer unto natural ones, inasmuch as these originate and flow from them, and serve as a foundation for the former."

To the Swedish clergymen who visited him a short time before his death, and who urged him to recant what he had written if it was not true, he replied, with great zeal and emphasis: —

"As true as you see me before you, so true is everything that I have written, and I could have said more had I been permitted. When you come into eternity you will see all things as I have stated and described them, and we shall have much to discourse about with each other."

Here, then, we have in this illustrious seer the unparalleled instance of a man, not in the enthusiasm of youth, but at the mature age of fifty-six years, standing among the first in the philosophical world, with reputation unsullied, high in office in his native country, with proffered promotion, giving up all, and proclaiming to the world that he was called by the Lord to the important office of revealing new truths of vast moment to his fellow-men—even the truths of a new dispensation, or of the second coming of our Lord and Saviour Jesus Christ.

Now, I appeal to you, one and all, Clergymen of the Christian Church, of every name, to obtain and read his writings. In the good Providence of the Lord, three among his most important works can be obtained without money and without price by the clergy and theological students of our country, by simply ordering them and sending the postage—as will be seen on the second page of the cover of this pamphlet.

Swedenborg does not require or desire you to believe anything contained in his writings on his simple declaration, but you are to believe the statements made, and doctrines proclaimed, in his writings, only as you perceive them to be true, and in strict accordance with the Sacred Scriptures. What have you to lose by reading his writings? Thousands of laymen and clergyman testify to you that they have found the greatest help and strength from reading them, even where they may not have read enough to fully recognize his claims.

Canon Wilberforce, of Southampton, England, one of the most distinguished clergymen of the English Church, visited this country a few years ago; and while he was here, being a prominent temperance man, the National Temperance Society gave him a reception, during which some one introduced me to him as a believer in the writings of Emanuel Swedenborg. Stopping a moment, and looking steadily at me and those in the immediate vicinity, he exclaimed, most emphatically: "Emanuel Swedenborg has done the Christian Church an immense service! an immense service!! especially in his explanation and illustration of the doctrine of the Lord. " These words were spoken manfully and boldly in the presence of members and clergymen of his own and other Churches. The doctrine of the Lord is the chief corner-stone of the New Jerusalem now descending from God out of Heaven. Let that doctrine be accepted by our Churches, and their creeds, so far as they are based on a tri-personal God, will need no revision; they will disappear.

"All things, " says a great authority, "are of God, who hath reconciled us to Himself by Jesus Christ, and hath committed unto us the ministry of reconciliation; to wit, that God was in Christ reconciling the world unto Himself, not imputing their trespasses unto them. " (2 Cor. v: 18, 19)

The late Professor George Bush and a large number of distinguished scholars and clergymen, after a most thorough and careful examination of Swedenborg's writings, assure us that in them they find the truths of a New Dispensation, even of the Second Coming of the Son of Man in the clouds of heaven. The light of a New Day is shining. Christian brethren, will you close your eyes against it?

Was there ever any greater need of a new revelation from God to teach men anew that, if they would reach heaven and happiness, they must repent and shun evils as sins against God, and strive to live a life according to the commandments? Look at the fearful evils which prevail in our beloved country; the love of rule, civil and ecclesiastical; the miserly love of money, selfishness, vanity and sensualism, in their worst and most degrading forms! Customs and habits prevail which threaten the extinction of at least the Protestant portion of the community in large sections of our country. A Catholic bishop stated, a few years ago, that one quarter of the inhabitants of New England are Catholics, and that one-fourth of the population give birth to 70 per cent. of the children born in New England. More recent inquiries, it is stated, show that the average number of children in a family among the Canadian French settled in New England, averages 5; whereas among the native New Englanders the average number of children in a family is 1-1/2. It is not difficult to see by whom the land of the Puritans will be ruled within the next quarter of a century. Seventy years ago, the average number of children to a family among New Englanders was fully equal to the number among the French to-day. Why this change? Fashionable habits of dress—tight lacing, which is worse to-day than ever before—has, to a large extent, destroyed the ability of the New England and other native American women to bear healthy and well-developed children, and to properly nurse them after they are born. Among our present deformed women, child-bearing is attended with much more danger and suffering than among well-developed, symmetrical, and beautifully formed women. No man who desires peace, health, and happiness in his home, and desires to leave children behind him, and to thus perform the most important use which can be performed in this life, should ever think of marrying a small-waisted woman.

Then again, to have a good family of children is thought not to be fashionable, among those who are led by fashion, as it interferes too much with one's selfish pleasures, they think; most dearly do they pay in after life, if they live many years, for their folly. Children are a blessing; and yet the most unnatural and injurious measures are adopted to prevent bearing children, even to the destroying of the unborn. The Catholic Church, through the confessional, holds some restraint over Catholics; but what restraint do our Protestant Churches hold over their members in regard to such evils? Look at the miserable caricatures of the female form printed in our fashionable magazines, and even in our daily papers, and sent forth and freely spread before our young girls, for them to pattern after, and thus deform themselves.

Look at the drunkenness, the leaden and congested faces of our steady drinkers of intoxicating drinks, and the innumerable deaths and the wretchedness and sorrow which follow such drinking; and remember that the chief support of such drinking at this day is the use of the drunkard's cup instead of "the fruit of the vine" as a communion wine in so many of our churches, and the example of so many of our clergy, backed up by the prescribing of such drinks by so many of our doctors. Do away with these two chief supports, and prohibition would be enacted and enforced throughout our land within five years.

Look at the use of tobacco, which is to-day recognized as one of the most deadly poisons, which when used by the young prevents the development of the human body, and at all ages causes innumerable diseases and deaths and an inability to withstand the encroachment of other causes of disease; and the smoke and saliva from the nostrils and mouths of those who use it, which are so unpleasant and disagreeable to those who are not accustomed to them, but who yet are so frequently compelled to breathe a polluted atmosphere. Please read the following and tell us whether to thus prevent the development of the body and lessen one's ability to withstand the causes of diseases should be shunned as a sin against God or not: —

Personal Experience of a Physician

SMOKING AND PHYSICAL DEVELOPMENT.

From the records of the senior class of Yale College during the Past eight years, the non-smokers have proved to have decidedly gained over the smokers in height, weight, and lung capacity. All candidates for the crews and other athletic sports were non-smokers. The non-smokers were 20 per cent. taller than the smokers, 25 per cent. heavier, and had 62 per cent. more lung capacity. In the graduating class of Amherst College of the present year, those not using tobacco have in weight gained 24 per cent. over those using tobacco, in height 37 per cent., in chest girth 42 per cent., while they have a greater average lung capacity by 8.36 cubic inches. —*Medical News.*

Just see the countenance which is given to this habit by too many of our clergymen—the example which they set! Yes, in many of our denominations, young men who are known to be smokers, or chewers of tobacco, with their breaths smelling of this filthy, poisonous weed, are deliberately licensed and ordained by Clergymen, when it is known that they will go in and out before young and old, setting them an example which will unquestionably do untold injury to the rising generation, and confirm old smokers and chewers in their injurious and destructive habits, and thus be instrumental in destroying many lives. What are the fathers and mothers in our churches thinking about when they consent to such an example being set before their children? Is it not time that they awake to the importance of choosing and introducing into office their own ministers, instead of entrusting this duty to the clergy? Swedenborg has given us the true signification of ordination by the laity. In speaking of the ordination of the Levites by the laity he says: "By the sons of Israel laying their hands upon the Levites was signified the transference of the power of ministering for them, and the reception of it by the Levites, thus separation. "—A. C. 10,023. It will be seen that it was not Aaron the priest who laid his hands upon the Levites when they were introduced into the office of the priesthood, but the laity, or the children of Israel; and we can all see how appropriate and significative the ceremony was; and it was strictly in accordance with republican usages of this day. It does not exalt the officer above the office which he fills.

Is there a race of men on earth to-day who stand in greater need of light on spiritual subjects, and of the services of good, earnest, clean, pure-minded Christian Missionaries, who shall call men and women to repentance, and by precept and example lead them to shun the fearful evils named above, and many others, as sins against God, more than the people of the United States? Look at our children, many of whom, if they live at all, grow up with crooked legs and spines, delicate muscles and irritable brains, imperfectly developed jaws and consequently crowded teeth, which commence decaying and torturing the young before they are twenty years old, instead of lasting during life as they should; all of which results principally from feeding children with starvation bread, or superfine flour bread, cakes, and puddings, instead of the "full corn in the ear, " or unbolted flour or meal, as the Lord has organized it in the kernel of grain. Many years ago scientific investigation demonstrated the fact that the portions of the grain which nourish the brain, muscles, and bones is principally confined to the dark, hard portion of the kernel immediately beneath the hull; this is not easily pulverized or rolled into superfine flour, and if it were the flour would not be white; but it goes principally into, the second and third runnings or as canal, shorts, and bran, and is fed to the horses, cattle, and hogs, causing them to be well developed, strong, and healthy, while our children, for the want of it, are half starved. Even a dog, it has been found by experiment, will starve to death on superfine flour bread, but will live well enough on Graham or unbolted flour bread. I have seen a child come near starving to death on such bread, and only rescued her from impending death by mixing mashed potatoes with the flour from which the bread was made. The little girl thought she could eat no other food but such bread, and if she ate anything else she threw it up. And yet, strange to say, I have known in one or more institutions under the care of physicians, which were devoted to the treatment of deformed and crippled children, superfine flour bread to be given them to eat.

It is fashionable and customary to use superfine flour bread; and as a physician, and an employer of men, I know how difficult it is to induce or persuade fathers and mothers, even for the sake of their children, to use Graham or unbolted flour bread, cakes, and puddings, which will give nourishment to the brain, muscles, teeth and bones, and all the fat and heat-producing material they need, instead of superfine white flour bread, cakes, and puddings, which give comparatively little more than fat and heat-producing material.

I remember very well when my wife and myself were traveling in Egypt up the Nile, and were at ancient Thebes, mounted on donkeys, going to the tombs of the kings, the young Arab girl, with a vessel of water upon her head, balanced by the ends of the fingers of one hand, who ran beside us over the sand, stones, and hills; for she was one of the most beautiful and symmetrical female forms I have ever seen. There was no contracted waist or humped shoulders, but a beautiful female figure, full of life, with splendid teeth and sparkling eyes. And on a visit to the house of our Arab dragoman, or guide, we saw how the flour or meal was made upon which that young girl was fed. In the court-yard two women were grinding at a mill as they ground thousands of years ago. There were two circular mill stones, perhaps 20 inches in diameter, standing in a basin; through the centre of the upper stone there was an opening through which the wheat was poured, and upon two sides were erect wooden handles, by which the women turned the stone round and round, and back and forth, and the meal escaped into the pan at the circumference. I said to our dragoman: "We have not had a bit of good bread in Egypt. We have been stopping at hotels where they think they must give the Americans and Englishmen white bread. Now, I wish you would bring me some bread made from that flour to-morrow morning; " and he brought us some bread, and it was by far the best bread that we had in Egypt.

The fearful evils which I have hastily named in the preceding pages, and many others which cause the prevailing deformities, diseases, insanity, and premature deaths, are not to be dragged along into the Church of the New Jerusalem now descending from God out of heaven; but our race is to be purified, renovated, and developed into a healthy, noble, symmetrical, graceful manhood by the new inflowing of truths from the Lord, pointing out the evils and falses which are causing the present suffering and wretchedness, and calling on men and women to shun such evils and falses as sins against God. A reformation from worldly motives is but "skin deep, " and generally only results in the changing of one bad habit for another. Men and women must be earnestly called to repentance, and to the absolute necessity of shunning the evils which prevent the development of the body, impair health and reason, and so fearfully shorten the average duration of human life, as sins against God, which will tell on their eternal destiny. The fact that individuals who drink intoxicating drinks, smoke or chew tobacco, or deform their bodies by tight dressing, sometimes live to old age under otherwise favorable circumstances, amounts to nothing. The simple question is, do such habits shorten the average duration of human life? If they do, they are a violation of the laws of God as manifested in the organization of the human body and in His Word.

CHAPTER VII.

THE WANTS OF THE CHRISTIAN CHURCH.

The Christian Church at this day, first of all, needs true doctrines which are in harmony with the Sacred Scriptures, and which all men who are willing to see and obey, using the reason with which God has endowed them, can accept and see to be true.

Second, such a law or principle of interpretation of the Sacred Scriptures, that when they are interpreted in accordance with it, every man and woman who is willing to see and obey the truth will find there is actually no conflict between the Word of the Lord and His works, and no real contradictions to be found in the Sacred Scriptures.

In the writings of Swedenborg the Lord has shown us that "all religion has relation to life, and that the life of religion is to do good; " and that, if we would enter into the heavenly life, or have heaven within us, we must strive faithfully and honestly to keep the commandments, not simply in external acts, but also in our motives, thoughts, and words, as well as in act. In the writings of Swedenborg the Lord has clearly revealed Himself and has come down to the comprehension of man—God in Christ and in His Word.

The Science of Correspondences enables us to see that the first eleven chapters of Genesis are purely allegorical, and in their spiritual and true sense treat of the regeneration of man, and his fall through the seduction of his lowest or sensual nature and appetites, as men are seduced to-day; and of a flood of evils and falses, similar to the flood which threatens to overwhelm the Christian world, at least in our land, at this day; and a New Church as an ark of safety. While the Science of Correspondences shows that there are no more contradictions in the Word of the Lord than in His works, there are apparent truths and real truths in both. It is an apparent truth that God is angry with the wicked every day; but the real truth is that God is never angry, but when man disobeys His laws and brings upon himself consequent suffering, it appears to him that God is angry. So it appears to us that night and darkness are caused by the going down of the sun, but the real truth is that the sun always shines and that night and darkness are caused by the earth's diurnal revolution on its axis. It will therefore be seen that if the Sacred

Scriptures are the Word of God and in accordance with His works, they must contain both apparent and real truths.

No man who has ever diligently and faithfully, without prejudice, read the Sacred Scriptures in the light of the Science of Correspondences, as revealed by the Lord through Emanuel Swedenborg, has ever failed to be satisfied that the Sacred Scriptures are Divine and plenarily inspired, and that they differ as much from the writings of men as do the works of God from the works of men. At this day, when so many of our clergy and intelligent laymen are beginning to doubt the special inspiration of the Sacred Scriptures, a knowledge of the Science of Correspondences, in accordance with which they were written, is wanted above every thing else, that the Christian Church "may revive again and draw breath through heaven from the Lord."

The Lord speaks to man in parables, and "without a parable," we read, "spake He not unto them." The Lord intimates in many passages that the Sacred Scriptures, or His words, contain a spiritual sense, as in the following: "It is the spirit that quickeneth; the flesh profiteth nothing; the words that I speak unto you, they are spirit and they are life." "The letter killeth, but the spirit giveth life."

"The early Christian Fathers, Clement of Alexandria, and Origen, understood that the Sacred Scriptures have a spiritual sense; and Origen—when that shrewd enemy of Christianity, Celsus, ridiculed the stories of the rib, the serpent, etc., as childish fables—reproaches him for want of candor in purposely keeping out of sight, what was so evident upon the face of the narrative, that the whole is a *pure allegory.*"—*Noble's Plenary Inspiration.*

"The idea of a spiritual sense in every part of the Scripture was the generally received doctrine of the Primitive Church—believed and taught by Origen, Ignatius, Justin Martyr, Jerome, Augustine, Pantaenus, Tatian, Theophilus, Pamphilius, Clement and Cyril of Alexandria, and nearly all the early Christian Fathers. And the same belief has been held by many eminent theologians ever since. Dr. Mosheim, speaking of the illustrious writers of the second century, says: 'They *all* attributed a double sense to the words of Scripture; the one *obvious* and *literal*, the other *hidden* and *mysterious*, which lay concealed, as it were, under the veil of the outward letter.' But the Fathers had no recognized rule for eliciting the spiritual sense. Each one's own spiritual perception was his only guide. A hundred different expositors, therefore, might give as many different expositions of the same text." — *Rev. B. F. Barrett.*

Every natural object is the form and embodiment of some spiritual idea or principle; and therefore it is the most perfect expression or type or picture of that idea.

"Inasmuch as the end of the creation is an angelic heaven out of the human race, and thus the human race itself, therefore all other things that are created are mediate ends, which being referable to man, look to these three things of man, his body, his rational part, and his spiritual part, for sake of conjunction with the Lord. For a man cannot be conjoined to the Lord unless he be spiritual; nor can he be spiritual unless he be rational; nor can he be rational unless his body is in a sound state. These things are like a house, of which the body is the foundation, and the rational is the house built upon it; the spiritual comprises those things which are in the house, and conjunction with the Lord is being at home in it."

Here are outlined clearly and distinctly three fields for much needed labor.

We see above, clearly taught by Swedenborg, that "a man cannot be spiritual unless he be rational, nor can he be rational unless his body be in a sound state." The reason is plain: for the natural corresponds to the spiritual; natural diseases and natural causes of disease correspond to spiritual diseases and spiritual causes of spiritual disease.

Swedenborg says that: "Diseases correspond to the lusts and passions of the mind; these, therefore, are the origins of diseases; for the origins of diseases in general are intemperance, luxuries of various kinds, pleasures merely corporal; also envyings, hatreds, revenges, lasciviousness, and the like; which destroy the interiors of man, and when these are destroyed the exteriors suffer and draw man into diseases, and thereby into death." — *Arcana Coelestia*, 5712.

For this reason, if a man is to be reformed and regenerated, his reformation must commence by his shunning natural falses and bad habits of life, which correspond to his spiritual evils.

Swedenborg's writings give us a wonderful insight into the causes and cure of both spiritual and natural diseases, as we shall hereafter see, and many suggestions which it would be well for us to heed. He says: —

"The man who is willing to be enlightened by the Lord, must take especial heed lest he appropriate to himself any doctrinal which patronizes evil; for man in such case appropriates it to himself, when he confirms it with himself, for thereby he makes it a principle of his faith, and still more so if he lives according to it. When this is the case, then evil remains inscribed on his soul and his heart; and when this effect has place, he cannot afterwards in any wise be enlightened by the Word from the Lord; for his whole mind is in the faith and in the love of his principle, and whatsoever is contrary to it, this he either does not see, or rejects, or falsifies." (A. C. 10,640.)

Every one can see how true this is in regard to evil habits which destroy health, reason, and life, such as the prevailing use of tobacco and the drinking of intoxicating drinks. If a man drinks thoughtlessly, without knowing any better, he can be taught and shown that it is wrong and a sin to drink poisonous fluids which are entirely unnecessary, and which endanger health, reason, life, and the welfare and happiness of all associated with him, and actually destroy vast multitudes of those who drink them moderately. All children and young persons who are free from bad examples and false teachings can be taught and can readily see that it is wrong and a sin to use such drinks; but let a man strive to justify such habits by the Sacred Scriptures, and to make them accord with his religious principles, and we all know how difficult it is for him ever to see the truth upon this and kindred subjects.

MUCH-NEEDED INSTRUCTION.

Inquiry should be made into the natural causes of disease, into which spiritual causes flow and cause the suffering, wretchedness, and premature deaths which prevail, and men and women should be led by precept and example to see them as evils and to shun them as sins against God. Swedenborg says: —

"Thus, by washing the feet, is meant to purify the natural principle of man; for unless this principle appertaining to man, when he lives in the world, is purified and cleansed, it cannot afterwards be purified to eternity; for such as the natural principle of man is when he dies such it remains; for it is not afterwards amended, inasmuch as it is that plane into which interior things, which are spiritual, flow in—it being their receptacle; wherefore when it is perverted, interior things, when they flow in, are perverted like it. " (A. C. 10,243.)

There are two great hindrances to the reformation of the world at this day; the first is false teaching in regard to evils, by which unlawful indulgences are justified, and in moderation held to be good; for by this the individual is strongly confirmed in their favor and prevented from seeing the truth. The second is the love of the evil which the truth condemns, which closes the mind against the truth, and, as it were, binds and imprisons the individual (see A. C. 5096). It must be self-evident to every intelligent Christian that if it is wrong to deliberately appropriate falses and evils "temperately" or moderately to the building up of our spiritual organizations, it is equally wrong to appropriate temperately those natural substances which correspond to falses and evils in a vain attempt to build up healthy natural bodies. Total abstinence in both cases is the only law of life. The lover of intoxicating drinks can never be radically reformed or regenerated until he resolves, with the help of the Lord, to stop drinking intoxicating drinks and sets himself honestly about it; so the thief must stop stealing, the vain woman must stop her tight dressing and habits of idleness; and so of all other evils affecting physical and spiritual health and life.

But to-day the great difficulty is, that multitudes of the young and of all ages become "bond-servants" to evil habits, which impair health and reason and shorten life, through ignorance, hereditary inclination, and the bad example of others. And how are they to regain their freedom, and the innocent to be protected from contamination and from a like slavery? The truth can alone make them free; and even when received by the willing and obedient, line upon line and precept upon precept may be required. And they will often have to endure many a hard struggle; and those who are free should have sympathy and charity, and judge them not. Men, women, and children must be taught that they have no right to follow habits which will endanger health and reason, and which observation and carefully collected statistics show will shorten the average duration of life; for to thus act is to violate the command, "Thou shall not kill. " The causes of ill health, deformity, and the prevailing insanity and premature deaths must be sought out and exposed, and a call to repentance must be made.

In the good providence of the Lord, we have men who, by education, diligent investigation, and careful observation, are most admirably adapted to give the needed instruction—physicians. Let physicians arm themselves with true doctrines, with the spiritual sense of the Word, with the Science of Correspondences and a knowledge of natural sciences, and they will be able to combat the prevailing evils as no other men can; and they should lead in all the great necessary reforms of this age that have regard to physical health, life, and morals. In almost every society of our Churches of any size will be found one or more medical men who have devoted their lives to the study of anatomy, physiology, the causes of disease, diseases and their cure, and the effects of poisons and the bad habits of dress, and other habits injurious to health; and they are able to speak with authority in regard to the prevailing evils of life, which are so destructive to our race. These men, thus providentially prepared, should be called into the field as lecturers. There is not a religious society which does not actually need the services of such teachers; and we can send no other missionaries to those outside of our church organizations who will, to the same extent, command their attention and respect. In order that the body with its environment may be a fit dwelling place for the Spirit, there are provided—

"*Uses for sustaining the body*, comprising its nourishment, clothing, habitation, recreation and enjoyment, protection and conservation of state. The uses created for the nourishment of the body comprise all things of the vegetable kingdom which are good for food and drink; fruits, berries, seeds, pulse, and herbs; all things of the animal kingdom which serve for meat, oxen, cows, calves, deer, sheep, kids, goats, lambs; not to mention milk; also fowls and fish of many kinds. " (D. L. W. 331.)

"Good uses, " says Swedenborg, "are from the Lord, and evil uses are from hell. Evil uses were not created by the Lord, but they originated together with hell. " (D. L. W. 336.) Among the evil uses he enumerates all kinds of poisons—in a word, "all things that do hurt and kill men. " (*Ibid*. 339.) Here, then, is a criterion by which we must judge of the suitability of any article for nourishing and supplying the wants of our natural bodies. It should be evident to every one that substances which have their origin from hell, which, when used as we use legitimate articles of food and drink, seriously endanger, hurt, and kill men, should never be used for such purpose.

Who are better qualified to judge as to what are evil uses than the physician, who has made them the study of his life? The men and women who are violating the laws of life cannot see that such violations injure them; for such violations palliate the sufferings which they cause, and make the transgressors feel better every time they indulge. The true physician, by precept and example, is qualified to lead all who are willing to be led to a higher life and to protect the innocent and the young.

That such teachers are most important at this day is manifest "from the signification of physicians as denoting preservation from evils— the evils which obstruct conjunction. In the Word, physicians, the art of physic and medicine, signify preservation from evils and falses.... That in the Word, physicians, the art of physic and medicine, signify preservation from evils and falses, is manifest from the passages where they are named.... Hence it is evident what *medicine* signifies, viz., that which preserves from falses and evils; for when the truth of faith leads to the good of love, it preserves, because it withdraws from evils." (A. C. 6502.)

Here, then, we have the men suitable for this use. Shall we call them into the fields which are ripe and ready for the harvest?

A clergyman who has a knowledge of the medical profession and of medicine, in speaking of the importance of such teachers, says: "Moreover, from their relation to the sick and suffering, from their habit of analyzing the mental and moral states of their patients, and from the deep, tender sympathy which sincere, God-fearing physicians have for suffering human beings, they are placed in a much closer relation to the people than any other vocation could give them. How many persons have been comforted, strengthened, instructed, and turned to uprightness of life through the kindly ministrations of their physicians!"

And church organizations are languishing for the want of such teachers, and can never thrive in true doctrine and good lives, as they should, without them.

Surely every one can but see of what immense benefit such lecturers would be, especially to the young in our churches. One physician might be employed by and serve several societies, giving to the different societies once or twice a week a lecture in each society, fully illustrated by drawings, plates, stereoscopic and microscopic views, which would attract young and old, and fill our churches to overflowing with those who now attend no church; and the latter, when they found a physician, with the consent of the church, thus clearly pointing out the great evils of life which cause so much suffering, wretchedness, sorrow, and so many premature deaths, and calling young and old, from a religious standpoint, to shun them as sins against God, could but feel that our churches are striving to elevate humanity, and are a great blessing, and that it would be desirable to belong to them, and especially to have their children brought up under the influence of the Church.

Nearly the same could be said in regard to the important services which a second class of teachers of which I am about to speak could render. By the lectures of the two new life would be infused into our churches, and they would stand upon a sure foundation by manifesting love to God and man in our external natural lives, by teaching and leading men to act from spiritual motives, and to be willing to see their evils, and to commence by shunning well-known evils as sins against God. What a glorious day would this open up to our churches and for the elevation of our race through them!

THE SECOND CLASS OF TEACHERS REQUIRED.

Physicians as teachers in our churches should have for a special work the teaching of truth as to the physical life of man in connection with his spiritual life—the laws of health, the causes of prevailing diseases, deformities, insanities, and premature deaths, together with the methods and the duty of shunning them as sins against God. But there are other evils and questions which require careful consideration in our churches, such as the true relation, according to the laws of justice, mercy, and right, which should exist between men as neighbors, citizens, and Christians; and the clear light of this New Day should be brought down to guide men into a life of peace and harmony and good-will in this wilderness state of the world. Important questions are pressing for a solution, and for a careful consideration, by the religious teachers of our churches, such as the ecclesiastical and civil government best adapted for men of different countries and races, especially for our own country and churches; the relation of capital and labor; the right of single individuals to hold an unlimited amount of real estate, and transmit it to their children; the rights of corporations and of women; and our duties to others in all the relations of life. Fortunately, we have in our churches legal men or lawyers, who, while familiar with the doctrines of the Church, have devoted their lives to the consideration of such questions. It would not be difficult to point out several members of the legal fraternity belonging to our church organizations who would be able to perform a great use to the Church as lecturers and acting as missionaries among those who do not attend church as opportunity may offer. They would enter into a field of usefulness almost altogether beyond the reach and influence of our present ministers. Their advice, their counsel, their discourse, in their legal practice, are channels for the introduction of Christian thought and doctrine otherwise closed. There is one passage in the Writings which indicates this use: —

"*And strengthen the things which remain that are ready to die*—that hereby is signified; that the things which pertain to the moral life should be vivified, appears from the signification of strengthening, as denoting to vivify the moral life by truths; *for truths from the Word vivify that life*, which, when it is vivified, is also strengthened, for it then acts as one with the spiritual life." (A. E. 188.)

To meet and vivify the moral life of man with truths from the Word is a use eminently adapted to the position and mind of the legal profession. We need the services of such ministers, especially at this day, when we inherit from the fallen churches of the past an inclination to the love of spiritual and temporal dominion or rule, and the love of money and of vain show without regard to use. The evils that result from the gratification of such perverted affections must be fearlessly exposed, and a call to repentance made, before the injustice, oppression, and wrong which exist all over the world can be materially lessened. Lawyers, by making a special study of the Word in connection with their professional-studies, could not fail to impart much valuable instruction both to the Church and the world.

Christian physicians and lawyers would take hold of men in their present low state, showing them what acts are evil and wrong, and why they are so; and would call on them to repent and stop doing the evil acts which the truth condemns, fully realizing that a man must cease doing evil before he can cease thinking and willing evil; or, in other words, that reformation must commence on the natural plane, and from the highest motives of which the individual at present is susceptible.

It is the duty of our clergy to teach spiritual truths and the spiritual sense of the Word, and to lead men and women to live good lives, in obedience to the Divine commandments, from spiritual and celestial motives. But it is difficult for them to fill the entire field where religious instruction is needed, for we are living in the midst of the most direful evils of life, which must be put away before the New Jerusalem can descend and have an abiding place with men. Evils so terrible as to destroy vast multitudes of men and women of all ages, and even innocent children, all around us, too frequently go unheeded by our clergy and the periodicals under their charge. I know that in this respect there are some noble exceptions among our clergy and editors; but however willing and anxious they may be, it is impossible for one man to possess the knowledge and to impart all the necessary instruction as perfectly as three men thoroughly educated and trained for the different fields for labor could do it.

To recapitulate: The physicians are required to teach and to lead men to obey, from a principle of obedience, the spiritual and natural laws of health and life; the lawyers are required to teach and lead men by spiritual truths to act from a principle of justice, truth, and neighborly love in all their relations with others; our ministers are required to teach and lead men to act from love to the Lord and thence the neighbor, and to do right because it is right, and to administer the ordinances of the Church.

While some church organizations are laboring earnestly for the reform of men and women addicted to evils, and are striving to guard the innocent and young; and while in many of the churches in England they are organizing their temperance societies and "Bands of Hope, " many of our organizations are as silent as the grave in regard to these evils. Can our churches prosper without teachers who are able to point out the evils of life which are so destructive to our race, and who are sufficiently free themselves to be able earnestly and consistently to call men to repentance, and to lead them to live orderly lives?

Various denominations of Christians, in sending forth missionaries to distant lands, have, of late years, been sending, among others, some well-educated physicians as missionaries, and have found them very efficient in reaching and influencing the people among whom they labor. May not all take a hint when some of the religious organizations around us are beginning to see the advantages of sending out medical missionaries? If we would reach the Gentiles, or non-church goers, in our midst, should we not follow their example? A vast number of children and young people are growing up in our country, who are more ignorant of the spiritual and natural laws of health and life than many in Gentile lands; many of them rarely read or hear the Sacred Scriptures read, and do not even know the Ten Commandments.

CHAPTER VIII.

METHODS FOR RESTRAINING AND CURING SPIRITUAL AND NATURAL DISEASES.

As there is a correspondence between the natural and spiritual causes of disease, so there must be a correspondence between the methods of restraining and curing natural and spiritual diseases.

First: Spiritual diseases or evils are restrained by punishments which, by force, as it were, counteract the inclination to do evil; corresponding to this method we have the Antipathic method of restraining natural diseases, which is one of the prevailing methods; for instance, for constipation cathartics are given, for a diarrhoea astringents, and opiates are given to forcibly relieve or restrain the symptoms of disease. Every one can but see that such remedies for the cure of natural diseases, like punishments for the cure of spiritual diseases or evils, are but palliative; for the reaction, if reaction ensue, is not in the right direction. It is true that a cure sometimes results in spite of the treatment, especially in transient cases, the vital forces restoring health during the temporary restraint of the diseased action; but in many cases the constipation is only aggravated by cathartics, and diarrhoeas are not benefited by astringents; and the evil man often becomes more vicious after punishment.

Second: Spiritual evils are often restrained by exciting one passion to restrain evil acts in another direction; for instance, acquisitiveness and vanity are often excited to restrain evil men from evil acts, which might result from hatred and a desire for revenge, thus calling off the attention from the prevailing evil inclination. Corresponding to this method of restraining spiritual diseases we have the Allopathic method of restraining diseased action in one organ by exciting diseased action in another organ or part, as is done when a cathartic is given for disease of the head or lungs, or when a blister is applied to the skin in case of internal diseased action; thus, as it were, calling off the attention of the vital forces from the diseased structures, and thus palliative relief is often obtained in natural as in spiritual diseases.

Third: Either from afflictions, suffering, disappointments, or from voluntarily hearkening to the truth, a man begins to feel a desire to change his life, and looking to the Lord he repents and resolves to obey the Divine Commandments by shunning evils as sins against God. But when he commences to do this, evil spirits flow into his mind and tempt him to again do evil acts; if the temptations are too strong he falls, but he may fall to rise again; he will either do this by renewing his resolution to overcome the evil inclination, or he will fall to rise no more, and keep on in his old course of life, perhaps worse than before. Thoughts come before actions; if a man, when tempted to do evil, resists the thoughts of doing the evil acts, every one can see that he is striking a blow at the perverted affection through which he has been tempted to do evil; consequently the step toward a cure is far more radical and permanent than it would have been if he had done the evil act.

Children and the young should be taught that to violate the Divine Commandments is a sin against God, and that they should resist their hereditary or acquired inclination to speak wrong words or do evil acts the moment such inclinations are manifested in their thoughts, which is far better than to allow them to move them to do evil acts. The cure of spiritual diseases by the resisting of temptation is a genuine method of cure. Corresponding with this for the treatment of natural diseases, we have their treatment by the use of Homoeopathic remedies. Only spirits of a similar inclination can tempt a man to do an evil act and thus manifest his unsubdued inclination to him, which enables him to see and overcome the inclination by resisting it. So, on the natural plane, it is only a poisonous substance or remedy, which is capable of causing a similar disease to the one existing, which can manifest the disease to the vital forces and thus enable them to react against the disease. But if the dose of the remedy given is too large it will aggravate the disease, as a cathartic dose of a cathartic remedy will aggravate a diarrhoea; but the vital forces may react and overcome the disease, or they may not, and the disease continue even worse than before. It is the reaction of the vital forces that overcomes the diseased action and effects the cure, and not the remedy, any more than it is the evil spirit that tempts man that overcomes his spiritual evils during regeneration. As it is not necessary that the temptation should be so strong as to make a man take the first step toward performing an evil act, to enable him to resist it if he will the moment the inclination is seen in his thoughts, so it is not necessary that a dose of a Homoeopathic remedy should be so strong as to aggravate the natural diseased action in the slightest degree before it can be seen by the vital forces, and a reaction follow. The size of the dose must be determined by experience; but we know that its effects need only to equal the effects of temptations which proceed no further than the thought of doing evil before reaction may follow, therefore we can form no conception of the minuteness of the dose which may be sufficient for a cure to follow.

But if a man would be restored to spiritual health by getting rid of his hereditary and acquired inclinations to do evil, he must acknowledge the Lord, diligently search His Word, and be willing to see and obey His commandments, which are the laws of spiritual health and life, and must be obeyed conscientiously, in intention, thought, word, and deed, if health is to be restored; otherwise, punishment, hope of reward, and temptations can only afford palliative relief at best. So in regard to natural diseases. If a man would be restored to physical health by getting rid of his hereditary and acquired inclinations to diseases, he must recognize that the laws of nature are the laws established for his good by the Lord, and he must diligently study the laws pertaining to health and life, and be willing to see and obey those laws as to sunlight, air, exercise, clothing, and in eating and drinking, etc., if he would be restored to health; otherwise, antipathic, allopathic, and even homoeopathic remedies will prove only palliative at best. If we expect to be well, spiritually or naturally, we must strive to know and obey the laws of health and life.

Temptations by evil spirits permitted and controlled by the Lord for the sake of removing many spiritual evils, and a corresponding action of homoeopathic remedies administered by a skillful hand, for the sake of removing natural diseases, are curative methods which belong to the New Jerusalem Dispensation, now descending from God out of heaven, making all things new—the Church of the future.

CHAPTER IX.

PERSONAL EXPERIENCE CONTINUED—AND EFFORTS.

Soon after I commenced reading the writings of Emanuel Swedenborg, while residing in Detroit, I was invited to attend a social gathering at the residence of one of the members of the congregation of believers in his writings in that city. During the evening, to my astonishment, fermented wine was passed around to the guests, of which quite a number partook. As already stated in the preceding pages, while a young man, through the efficient teachings of Baptist and Congregational clergymen and prominent members of the churches, and the results of drinking which I witnessed, I was providentially enabled to see that to use drinks which endangered health, reason, and life was wrong, and consequently a sin; and with many others I signed a pledge never to drink intoxicating drinks during health. The reader can imagine how I was shocked to see intoxicating wine presented and partaken of among gentlemen and ladies who professed to be receivers and believers in a new revelation of Divine truth from God to man. I immediately saw the clergyman of the society, and asked him if Swedenborg teaches that it is right and proper to drink an intoxicating wine. He replied that he did.

He and members of his society were holding Sunday afternoon meetings for the purpose of reading the writings and discussing such questions as might arise, which meetings I attended. I said to the reverend gentleman that I would like to have this wine question discussed at our next meeting, to which he assented. At that meeting, I brought up the medical and scientific aspects of the question, and endeavored to show that fermented wine was a dangerous poison, it having destroyed vast multitudes of the human race, and that it performed no use when taken into the stomach of healthy men and women; and, consequently, that it is wrong to drink a wine which does so much harm. The clergyman tried to justify its use by quoting certain comparisons which Swedenborg had made between the apparent combat which takes place during fermentation and the combat which ensues during the regeneration of man, and the clearness of resulting wine after fermentation and that of truth in the mind after regeneration, and also of the purity of alcohol after it has been through certain processes, which he named, compared with pure truth.

But we know that pure alcohol cannot be used as a beverage, and therefore it is certain that these comparisons were simply as to the clearness of fermented wine after fermentation, and the purity of alcohol after being purified; and that they have nothing to do with the inherent quality of these fluids, or their ability to affect man when he drinks them. We had an earnest discussion of the question from our different standpoints, but neither of us was satisfied with the result; and, consequently, we adjourned the discussion of the subject until the next Sabbath afternoon. In the meantime, the clergyman prepared a discourse, which he delivered on Sunday morning, in which he endeavored to show that fermentation was caused by an influx of angels from the highest heaven into the juice of the grape, stirring it up and cleansing it from "inherent impurities. " Providentially, during the week, I had obtained a copy of Swedenborg's work on the "Angelic Wisdom Concerning the Divine Love and Wisdom, " in which he teaches that all poisonous substances which do harm and kill man derive their life from or through hell. When we came together in the afternoon to discuss the question, we were about as far apart as it was possible to be, as the reader can readily see. He took the ground that fermentation was caused by influx from the highest heaven, and I took the ground that it was caused by influx from the lowest hell, and we had an earnest discussion; but he certainly did not satisfy me nor many of his audience, if any, that his position was true. How could he? for there is no doubt but that fermented wine has harmed and killed more of the human race in ages past than any other poison. As a result of that discussion, within my knowledge, fermented wine was never again used at the sociables of that society during my residence in Detroit.

Within perhaps a year after that discussion, I was baptized and united with the Detroit Society of the New Church. When I came to understand, from the writings of Swedenborg, the true signification of water and the ordinance of baptism—that water signified natural truth and that baptism introduced one into the Church, and signified that man is to be regenerated or purified by living a life according to the truth, and that the head represented the man—I did not regard immersion as so important as I had previously, consequently I was baptized by the application of water to the head. There is, I think, no serious objection to any one being baptized by immersion who prefers it. Children should, I think, be baptized into the Church, and be brought up to feel that they belong to the Church, and are expected to live the life of the Church. More and more have I seen the importance of bringing children up under the influence of the

Church, where they should be instructed and entertained and thus kept away from bad company.

WHY A SEPARATE NEW-CHURCH ORGANIZATION.

Swedenborg made no attempt to organize the believers in the revelations made by the Lord through his instrumentality into a separate church organization, and nowhere in his writings does he express the opinion that such a separate organization would ever be needed or desirable. And he apparently expected that the prevailing false doctrines of the churches would, in the increasing light of the New Jerusalem, be seen to be false by the clergy of existing church organizations; and that through them the laity would be enabled to see that they are false, and thus they would be put away, as is manifest in passages which I have quoted elsewhere; also see T. C. R. 784.

When individual men or churches put away false doctrines, they are prepared, if in the good of life, to see and receive the truth; consequently Swedenborg says that although the First Christian Church has come to its end through false doctrines and evils of life, yet it is to revive again through the instrumentality of the newly revealed science of correspondences; consequently it is not to utterly perish, for there is a remnant within its borders.

Then the reader will inquire, "Why was an external New-Church organization ever formed? " We have not to look far to find the reason. First, there was a vast multitude of intelligent men and women who did not belong to any church organization, and when some of them came to see and believe the new doctrines, they naturally desired to be baptized and to join a church organization; but seeing clearly in the light of the new revelations that, according to the Sacred Scriptures, God is one in essence and in person, and that that one God was manifested to man in the person of the Lord Jesus Christ, and that He made that human form Divine and is henceforth to be worshiped as one God in His Divine Humanity, and that a life according to His sayings and the commandments is essential to salvation, they could not join the prevailing churches, for they could not assent to their creeds.

Second. When, as soon occurred, both clergymen and laymen, belonging to various church organizations, began to read the writings, and to see that the Lord is in very deed now coming in the clouds of heaven, and desired to let the new light shine among their brethren, they found that they were often not free to do so without giving offense; and in not a few instances clergymen found that they were silenced as preachers, and sometimes both clergymen and laymen were expelled, for believing the Heavenly Doctrines instead of the creeds; consequently the receivers of the doctrines of the New Dispensation had no choice but to form a new church organization. But at this day there is a vast change, and I trust that from but a very few if any church organizations would a lay member be expelled for believing in the Supreme Divinity of the Lord Jesus Christ, and that the Sacred Scriptures are Divine and plenarily inspired, and that a life according to the Lord's sayings and His Commandments is essential to salvation. Consequently there are thousands of earnest receivers of the Heavenly Doctrines of the New Jerusalem scattered throughout the various churches, gradually leavening, as I trust, the whole lump; and there are clergymen not a few who are gradually beholding, with more or less fullness, the light of this New Day; and as they receive it, large numbers of them are not slow to let the light shine among their fellow-men, as they are prepared to receive it.

The Lord has given to men freedom and reason, and they are responsible for their acts. To whom do a clergyman and members of a church organization owe fealty, to the Lord and His Word and the members of the congregations where they worship, or to a creed and church or a church organization formulated and organized during darker ages of the world and Church? Should men or should they not, when they behold the glorious light of the Lord's Second Coming in the clouds of heaven, stand in their place and proclaim the glad tidings to all who are willing to hear?

Swedenborg, in giving the spiritual sense of the second chapter of the Apocalypse, in No. 69 of the *Apocalypse Revealed*, says: —

"This and the following chapter treat of the seven churches, by which are described all those in the Christian Church who have any religion, and out of whom the New Church, which is the New Jerusalem, can be formed; and this is formed by those who APPROACH THE LORD ONLY, AND AT THE SAME TIME PERFORM REPENTANCE FROM EVIL WORKS. The rest, who do not approach the Lord alone, from the confirmed negation of the divinity of His humanity, and who do not perform repentance from evil works, are indeed in the Church, but have nothing of the Church in them."

Personal Experience of a Physician

If all clergymen and members of our churches, the moment they begin to see that portions of their creeds are false and injurious in their tendency, instead of trying, by proclaiming the truth among their brethren, to have the false doctrines removed and true doctrines substituted, were to immediately forsake the church organization in which, in the good providence of the Lord, they stand, what hope would there be for the perpetuation of existing churches as Christian organizations at all? The great danger at this day is that false doctrines will be seen faster than true doctrines will be seen to take their place, and thus our churches and members will be left desolate and return to a Gentile state. For instance, if our clergy and intelligent laymen begin to see, as many of them seem to be doing already, that the doctrine of a tri-personal God, instead of a trinity in unity, and the doctrine of the vicarious atonement are contrary to the teachings of the Sacred Scriptures, and unreasonable and inconsistent, and do not at the same time see clearly the scriptural doctrine that God is one in essence and in person, and that in the person of our Lord Jesus Christ that one God was manifested for the purpose of reconciling the world unto Himself, such individuals are almost sure sooner or later to deny the Divinity of the Lord Jesus Christ, and that the Sacred Scriptures are divine and special revelations from God to man, and consequently plenarily inspired.

The doctrines which are false in the prevailing church organizations must go—they are going—from the minds of their members if not from their creeds. Then are these organizations to become Gentile and stand like the remnants of the Ancient Church, which we behold in southern and eastern Asia? I think not; for we are told, as has been already stated in the revelations made by the Lord through Emanuel Swedenborg, that the science of correspondences was revealed that the Christian Church "may revive and again draw breath from the Lord through heaven. " Gentiles received the Lord at His first coming with joy; and so I believe the Gentiles in and out of our church organizations will receive Him now as He comes in the clouds of heaven. In the light manifested in the Sacred Scriptures by the aid of the science of correspondences, every willing and obedient man and woman is able to see that God is one, and that the Lord Jesus Christ, or God in His Divine Humanity, is that one God and the only Being whom men should and whom angels do worship. Then of what unspeakable importance it is that the attention of all clergymen and laymen be speedily called to the writings for the

Church of the New Jerusalem which is now descending from God out of heaven!

After practicing medicine for ten or twelve years, and on accepting the chair of "Theory and Practice of Medicine" tendered by the Western Homoeopathic College at Cleveland, Ohio, I commenced, as it were, the study of the practical department of my profession anew, in order to prepare myself for filling the chair profitably to the students and creditably to myself. While preparing forgiving lectures, and especially in after years while away from my active medical practice at Detroit, giving a course of lectures at Cleveland every winter, I began to study and investigate in my leisure hours the causes of diseases. Step by step I pursued my investigations, until I became satisfied that most of the deformities, diseases, and insanity which exist have been caused by the violation of the physical and spiritual laws of our being which could have been avoided in the past, and which can and must be in the future, if our race is to be restored to a state of healthy, symmetrical, and noble manhood. Consequently I came to the conclusion that it is far more important that men, women, and children should be taught the laws of health and to understand the causes of the prevailing deformities and diseases, and how to shun them, than it was for them and their children to get sick, deformed, and suffer, and often to pay their hard-earned money to doctors for the uncertain chance of being cured—in fact, that "an ounce of prevention is worth more than a pound of cure."

As a result of my investigations I wrote a series of articles for the *Detroit Tribune* on the bad habits which cause diseases, insanity, and deformity; and, as opportunity offered, I gave lectures upon such subjects; and finally I wrote a work entitled the "Avoidable Causes of Disease," of 348 pages, of which I printed several editions, the first of which was in 1859, and furnished to different publishers, and advertised to a limited extent; after that it was published for several years by Messrs. Mason Brothers, of New York; after which it came into my hands again. I also wrote a pamphlet of 48 pages on "Marriage and its Violations," which, for a time, was bound separately, but afterward was bound with the "Avoidable Causes of Disease." In all, eleven editions of the work have been printed; the last edition was printed by Messrs Boericke & Tafel, of Philadelphia, who will probably publish any future editions which may be demanded.

Personal Experience of a Physician

I soon found, what my publishers found after me, and other writers and their publishers have found, that it does not pay to advertise books which contain the greatest amount of practical and useful information which is calculated to benefit readers, especially if they call in question the bad habits and evils of life in which so many people indulge; consequently, feeling that a work treating of diseases and their cure, in which I could advertise my first work and call special attention to it, would sell more readily, I wrote a book of 404 pages, entitled "Family Homoeopathy, " in which I took great pains to carefully describe in few words the various diseases, and gave as definite and positive instruction as was practicable to guide laymen, so that harmless homoeopathic remedies might take the place of drastic drugs and injurious domestic remedies, which are so frequently used when it is thought not necessary to call a physician, or before his arrival when called. At the end of this volume I inserted a carefully prepared table of the contents of the "Avoidable Causes of Disease, " occupying three pages, and referred not unfrequently to that work when treating of various diseases.

With but very slight efforts, and no advertising on my part, "Family Homoeopathy" sold very well—principally through the different homoeopathic pharmacies in our country; and this increased the sale of "The Avoidable Causes of Disease" very materially, as I expected it would. Seventeen editions of "Family Homoeopathy" have been printed and sold, the last edition by Dr. E. R. Ellis, of Detroit, Michigan, who will continue to print and supply applicants as wanted.

SPIRITUAL CAUSES OF DISEASES.

As I continued my investigation into the causes of disease, and especially as I read the writings of Emanuel Swedenborg, I began to see more and more clearly that diseases, to a large extent at least, have a spiritual origin, and that the great obstacles to the removal of their causes lie in the false doctrines of Christian churches. When selfish men who were leaders in the churches desired to exercise their love of rule in spiritual and natural things and to exercise despotic power, when they desired to reduce other men to slavery and to hold them as slaves, or when they desired to gratify other perverted passions and sensual appetites, they all went to the Bible and strove to justify their conduct from its pages, with the expectation of reaching heaven at last; for this purpose it required the invention of special doctrines, and these they taught to their children, and thus the Word of God was made of no effect by the traditions and doctrines of men.

Unfortunately for the Protestant Church, early in its history, instead of "If ye would enter into life, keep the commandments, " there was substituted the doctrine of justification by faith alone; which led men, especially the young, to hope that by getting religion and having faith, they could at any time escape the legitimate penalties which are attached by the Lord to evil doing. No young man, religiously brought up, expects to go to hell; but he intends to repent and be converted before he dies; he often thinks he will "sow his wild oats" first, instead of earnestly and faithfully striving to keep the Divine commandments from his youth up. Evil thinking and doing develop an infernal life within him, which often gradually gains strength until he is ruled by his perverted appetites and passions; and day by day his ability to regain his freedom grows less.

When the priesthood of the Roman Catholic Church began to teach men that the punishment which rightly inheres to the doing of evil can be escaped by confessing to the priest, doing penance, and receiving absolution, and that every Catholic priest has from the Lord the power to forgive sins and to grant indulgences, then the hope of escaping the penalties of sin by something short of keeping the Divine Law in everyday life was held out to the young of the Catholic laity, similar to that which the doctrine of faith alone offered to the young of the Protestant world; and the results have been similar. We know, however, that among religious teachers there are many to-day in all of the various sects of Christians who have put away, or are gradually putting away, or materially modifying, the perverted doctrines of the past. As an illustration of the changes which are taking place, I clip the following from an English paper, recently received: —

"The Rev. T. Vincent Tymms, the new Principal of Rawdon College, preaching to his late congregation at Clapham, said: —

"'From the first day I stood in this pulpit until now, I have desired to tear away from every heart that obscuring veil of pagan thought which first attributes a wrathful justice to the Father and a tender mercy to CHRIST, and then represents the Son as dying to soothe the anger and satisfy the relentless demands of the Father. Such unholy and revolting ideas are the leaven of heathenism, not the unleavened bread of Christian truth. '

Personal Experience of a Physician

"This is from the first of 'Three Farewell Sermons, ' published by Messrs. James Clarke & Co., Fleet Street, E. C."

More and more, as time progressed, I began to realize that there was very little chance for any radical improvement of our race until the false doctrines which have come down to us from the dark ages were put away; and knowing that in the writings of Emanuel Swedenborg we have a new revelation from the Lord, even the truths of his Second Coming in the clouds of heaven, which are destined to make all things new by leading men back to a life of obedience to the Divine commandments; and, furthermore, believing the most important missionary field to-day in the world to be among the clergy of our country, I wrote an "Address to the Clergy" of 24 pages. This Address I sent to over 50,000 clergymen. A few years before I wrote that Address, the late Mr. L. C. Iungerich, of Philadelphia, through the book publishing firm of J. B. Lippincott & Co., of that city, had offered to clergymen who would order and send the stamps to pay the postage, Swedenborg's "True Christian Religion, " and afterward he added the "Apocalypse Revealed; " and the New Church Tract Society added to the above works "Heaven and Hell, "—all to be sent free to clergymen on receipt of postage. Several thousand copies of the above works had been sent when I wrote and sent out my Address. Upon the second page of the cover of my tract was a notice of the above-named gift books; and my aim was to hastily call the attention of clergymen to them, and to give them some idea of the claims of Swedenborg's writings to their attention, and to encourage them to send for and to read the books thus providentially within their reach. As a result of receiving the Address, thousands of clergymen sent for and obtained one or more of the above books.

When I commenced sending the above-named Address to the clergy, I resolved to devote one-tenth of my income to the work of spreading a knowledge of the doctrines of the New Jerusalem and of an orderly life among my fellow-men. I can truly say, and will say for the encouragement of others, that as I have given I have received; for never had I prospered financially as I have since that resolution was made and lived up to. After having secured a competency for myself and family I did not stop at one-tenth of my income.

The result of sending the Address was so satisfactory that I wrote and compiled a work of 260 pages, entitled, "Skepticism and Divine Revelation, " with the intention of sending it to the clergy. My aim was to present a hasty view of the application of the science of correspondences in the interpretation of the first chapters of Genesis, and some other parts of the Word, and to meet the arguments of skeptics, and thus to show that the Sacred Scriptures are Divine revelations from God to man, and plenarily inspired, consequently differing as much from the words of man as God's works do from the works of man. In that work the attention of the reader is called to the creation of the world, the creation of man and woman, Eve, the Garden of Eden, its trees and river, the fall of man, the serpent, Cain and Abel, the flood, Noah, Shem, Ham, and Japheth, the flood of waters, the Ark, the Tower of Babel, Sun worship and idolatry, spiritualism, the little reliance to be placed upon communications from spirits, and why. Next, the doctrines of the New Jerusalem— God, the Incarnation, the Divine Trinity, sacrificial worship, the Cross, a true and heavenly life, the end of the world and Second Coming of the Lord, the resurrection, state of infants in the other life, the state and condition of the Heathen and Gentiles in another life, the New Jerusalem—the Church of the Future—the Crown of all Churches, the Divine promise to those who receive the New Jerusalem at the Lord's Second Coming as revealed through Emanuel Swedenborg.

Such were the subjects discussed in the light of the revelations made by the Lord's chosen servant. My aim was to produce the best work I could. Consequently, when I found in the writings of others passages, or even whole sections, in which the ideas that I desired to present were as well or better conveyed than I thought I could present them, I selected them, giving the writers credit for the same, and the sixteenth and twenty-third chapters were written at my request by the Rev. William B. Hayden, who assisted me materially in seeing the work through the press. About one-half of the matter in the volume was selected from other writers.

I commenced to send this work in editions of 10,000 to the clergy of our country, and when I had sent about 50,000, I had the "Address to the Clergy" printed and bound with it, and both were sent to the Catholic clergy, to whom the Address had not previously been sent. From that time both works have been printed and bound in one volume. About 65,000 of the above works, containing a notice of the gift books, named in preceding pages, on the second page of the cover, have been sent to the clergy of America, about 10,000 have been sent to physicians, and as many more have been circulated

Personal Experience of a Physician

among laymen. The sending of this book to the clergy immensely increased the orders for the gift books.

The above works have been translated into the German language, and about 48,000 copies sent to German-speaking clergymen in Germany and other parts of Europe, and in our own country. They have been translated into the Swedish language, and about 6000 copies have been sent to the clergy of Sweden and Norway and circulated among the laity; and they have been translated into Italian, and 10,000 sent to and circulated in Italy. And more recently they have been translated into French, and 20,000 printed which are now being sent to the clergy of France and the French-speaking clergy of other European countries, and of our own country.

Then, I have aided materially in sending other works to the clergy of our country, either explaining or containing the doctrines of the New Jerusalem, upon the second page of the covers of which will be found a notice of the gift books offered to clergymen. I aided with money the Swedenborg Publishing Association in sending Rev. Mr. Ravlin's "Progressive Thoughts on Great Subjects" to all the clergy of our country whose names could be had; and, later, I have aided the American Swedenborg Printing and Publishing Society in sending, first, "The New Jerusalem and Its Heavenly Doctrines; " second, "The Doctrine of the Lord; " third, "The Doctrine of Life"—all three Swedenborg's own works—to all the clergy in our country whose names could be readily obtained; in all 82,500. So that almost every clergyman in our country has had an opportunity to acquire some knowledge of the doctrines and revelations made by the Lord through Emanuel Swedenborg for the benefit of men in this new age—doctrines very different from those formulated in the creeds of bygone centuries—and thousands of our clergy are beginning to realize, that we must return to the rational and plain doctrines taught in the Sacred Scriptures, and summed up by the Lord when on earth in the Two Great Commandments, Thou shalt love the Lord with all thy might and strength, and thy neighbor as thyself, and that we must commence the new life by repentance, or by being willing to see our evils and to shun them as sins against God.

As a result of the efforts made by others and myself to make known to the clergy the offer of the gift books, 32,831 clergymen have sent for and obtained "The True Christian Religion, " 30,887 have obtained "Heaven and Hell, " and 25,522 have obtained "The Apocalypse

Revealed, " according to the report of the Trustees of the Iungerich fund (May, 1891).

COMMUNION WINE.

For several years after I joined the Church I paid little attention to the subject of communion wine. But at last an article appeared in a New-Church paper, in which the writer claimed that fermented wine was a good and useful article to be used as a beverage, and he tried to justify its use by the teachings of the Church. Such views were so contrary to what I regarded as true, that I immediately commenced a more careful and critical examination of the writings of Swedenborg, to ascertain what is taught therein as to wine. I soon found that he distinctly recognized two kinds of wine, as does the Bible: one kind unfermented, a good and nourishing fluid to which he always gives a good signification when its use is not abused; and the other kind, known by its effects on man when he drinks it to be fermented, to which he has never given a good signification when it is clear from the context that reference is had to fermented wine. And I will here say that my opponents in the Church have done precisely what the advocates of slavery, intoxicating drinks, and skeptics have done in their appeals to the Bible to sustain their views. They find here and there a comparison and passage which, by placing their own construction upon them, they think will justify their views, while they totally ignore a large number of passages which most clearly and positively teach a totally different doctrine; and they ignore scientific facts, the well known effects of drinking fermented wine, and the testimony of ancient writers whenever such testimony does not accord with their own views. Thus they uphold the use of the drunkard's cup as a beverage and even as a sacramental wine; and within my knowledge more than one poor man in our Church who was struggling to reform his life has been led back by partaking of it to drunkenness.

A distinguished clergyman said in a letter to the writer: —

"I can never forget the experience already related to you when Mr. — —, my wife's brother-in-law, a gentleman of classical education, had become a sober man through my efforts and received the heavenly doctrines... Then came the Lord's Supper and we had fermented California wine. I handed him the cup, he drank, and after church he fled to some place where wine could be had, came home late in the evening drunk, and continued drinking for three months, until he died one evening after being brought home beastly drunk. Unfermented wine is no seducer, and had Mr. —— been given such in the Sacrament, he might be living, a sober man, to-day. Your books on the 'Wine Question' deserve, therefore, all that you have done and expended under the Lord's guidance for their publication and circulation, and God only knows how much good they will yet have to do."

Another clergyman wrote: —

"I was called to officiate at the funeral of a child. The parents—who were non-professors of religion—became much interested in the New Church. I furnished them suitable reading matter and visited them occasionally. Within a year they united with our Society. The man had formerly been a drinking man, but had ceased entirely. They were regular attendants on our church services. He was a mechanic. His well-behaved life restored public confidence in him, and he soon found constant employment at his trade. After about two years he felt a desire to take the Lord's Supper. I did not dissuade him; for, as he had abstained so long and faithfully, I felt sure he would continue. He presented himself with the communicants. Upon receiving the cup he took a sip and moved to return the cup to me; but suddenly, the old appetite being touched by the alcoholic spark, he returned the cup to his lips—it was about two-thirds full-and nearly drained it, as though urged on by demons. Poor man! Realizing what he had done, and evidently feeling disgraced, he at once arose and left the temple. From that time he returned to drink, and I have been unable to regain sufficient influence over him to effect his return to our services.

"Another man in my Society formerly drank to excess. I dare not encourage him to come to the communion. A majority of our members favor intoxicating wine for the Lord's Supper. How they can do so after witnessing its dreadful effects, I cannot understand. But the light is spreading, and may the Lord hasten the full day."

O Lord! how long? how long shall such evils continue in our churches?

Of course I replied to the article in the New-Church paper alluded to above, and others replied to me, and I to them in return; but it was not long before notice was given that the discussion would cease, and that with three unanswered articles against me in one number of the paper, and that in a paper edited by a clergyman, and published by the General Body of the Church. Well, looking for the welfare of the Church and its members which I loved, I could not stand still and see such false and dangerous views boldly and dogmatically proclaimed in the most extensively circulated periodical of the Church without doing my best to counteract them. Consequently I wrote a reply in a tract form, and sent it to every New-Churchman whose name I could obtain. This was but the beginning. An article appeared in another periodical of the Church to which I was allowed to reply; but the discussion was soon closed, and I was given no chance to reply to the last communication, and a reserved communication which was published afterward. Finding that there was no chance to present the temperance side of the wine question fairly before the readers of these two periodicals, I was led to write several pamphlets in reply to such articles as appeared in favor of the use of fermented wine, in which I endeavored to present fully and fairly, generally in the language of its advocates, their views of the question, and I endeavored to answer them in the light afforded by the Sacred Scriptures, the writings of the Church, ancient history, science, and well-known facts as to the manufacture and preservation of unfermented and fermented wines in all ages.

Several pamphlets were published in reply to the advocates for the use of fermented wine in our New-Church periodicals in the course of five or six years, of which about 10,000 of each were printed and sent to all Newchurchmen whose names I was able to obtain in this country, England, and elsewhere, hoping to reach as far as possible the readers of the writings of my opponents and others. The following are the names of the pamphlets written, printed, and sent, viz: "Pure Wine, Fermented Wine, and Other Alcoholic Drinks, " published in 1880; "The Wine Question in the Light of the New Dispensation, " in 1882; "Reply to the Academy's Review, " in 1883; "Intoxicants, Prohibition, and our New-Church Periodicals, " 1885, to which was added "Deterioration of the Puritan Stock, " 1884; making in all, with index, 736 pages.

Finally, I had printed an edition of all of the above pamphlets from the plates, and bound in cloth, of which I sent a copy to all New-Church ministers in the world whose names I could get, and to some others.

My controversy with the clergy on the wine question led me to fear that there were other evils gradually creeping into the Church

Personal Experience of a Physician

organization which should be exposed, and against which both laymen and clergymen should be warned; therefore, I wrote a tract entitled, "The New Church: its Ministry, Laity, and Ordinances, with an Appendix on Intoxicants and Our New-Church Periodicals, " published and sent out in 1886, the latter part to answer some articles which had recently appeared in the Church papers. This tract was sent to about 10,000 or 11,000 Newchurchmen.

Then I wrote and compiled and condensed from my previous writings, including "The Avoidable Causes of Disease, " a work of 511 pages, fully presenting the wine question in all its aspects, and the use of tobacco and opium, and the bad habits of women, faulty methods of rearing children, etc., etc., of which in paper covers I sent out over 10,000 to my New-Church brethren, and about 40,000 copies I sent to clergymen of various denominations.

In the year 1883 my attention was seriously called to the signs of deterioration of the Puritan stock in New England, especially in Massachusetts, my native State, where it was shown that in six years, ending in 1881, the deaths among the native population fully equaled, if they did not exceed, the births; whereas, among the people of foreign birth, the births exceeded the deaths by over 87,000. And I found, on visiting my native town in Western Massachusetts, and the school district where I attended, where we used to have about thirty scholars in the winter and twenty in the summer, when I was a boy, and although there are but two families less residing there now than when I was a boy, and all native Americans, still I found that they had but eight or nine scholars during the winter, and not enough to keep up a school in summer.

As a result of my inquiries I wrote a work of 52 pages, calling attention to the spiritual and natural causes of such decline of the native stock, and especially to the bad habits and false ideas of men and women which have produced it. This pamphlet I entitled, "Deterioration of the Puritan Stock, and its Causes, " and printed 140,000 copies, which I sent to all the clergymen and physicians in our country whose names I could get, regarding them as the teachers and leaders of the people, and largely responsible for the existence of at least some of the prevailing evils of life.

Within the last few years pamphlets have been written by prominent clergymen of some of the prevailing denominations advocating the use of fermented wine, especially for sacramental purposes, in strong language, and claiming that it is a good and useful fluid. This seemed to aid and comfort distillers, brewers, and saloonists very much. At last one appeared entitled "Communion Wine," in which the advocates for the use of the "Fruit of the Vine," or pure unfermented wine, were assailed in no very gentle language. Several thousand of this pamphlet were sent by a Rev. Doctor of Divinity to clergymen, with a special request from him, to at least some of them, that they should read them and give him their opinion as to its merits. About 285 clergymen responded, most of them in favor of the views contained in the pamphlet, but 22 most decidedly opposed. The arguments in favor of fermented wine were based upon assumptions which were entirely groundless, and which have again and again been exposed. I could but feel that the time had come when a concise statement of the truth upon the wine question should be written and placed in the hands of every clergyman in our country; and as, in the controversy extending over several years, I had had occasion to examine the wine question in all of its various aspects, and to read whatever I could find written on both sides of the question, and had had suggestions from, and the cooperation of, some of the most distinguished scholars upon this question in this country and England, I felt that it was my duty to write a reply, which I did, of 38 pages, which was printed in connection with a short article on "The Holy Supper is Representative," by Mr. J. R. Hoffer, editor of the Mount Joy *Herald*, Mount Joy, Pa. Of this pamphlet over 80,000 were sent by Mr. Hoffer to clergymen in the United States. And of my reply alone, in a tract form, which is based upon the letter of the Sacred Scriptures—the testimony of ancient writers and science—about 50,000 copies have been printed and distributed by Mr. J. N. Stearns, 58 Reade Street, New York, who keeps a supply on hand to fill all orders.

The last pamphlet before this one which I have written is one recently published by "The Swedenborg Publishing Association," of Germantown, Philadelphia, Pa., entitled "The Essential Points of the Wine Question Carefully Examined," which, with an Addendum of 6 pages by W. J. Parsons, son of the late Professor Theophilus Parsons, contained 70 pages. This pamphlet was written for Newchurchmen and based upon the Sacred Scriptures as unfolded by the Science of Correspondences revealed through Swedenborg. This pamphlet was sent only to 10,000 Newchurchmen.

Personal Experience of a Physician

THE RESULTS OF EFFORTS IN BEHALF OF TEMPERANCE.

The reader may reasonably inquire what results have followed all the efforts which I have made to call the attention of the clergy and laity of the New Church, and the clergy of other churches, to the importance of using as a communion wine, the genuine "Fruit of the Vine" as the Lord has organized, ripened, and sweetened it in the grape, instead of a leavened or fermented wine, which, when used as a beverage, causes disease, drunkenness, insanity, and death, in innumerable instances, among the clergy and laity of our churches, and enslaves their children often before their rational faculties are fully developed. I am happy to say that to-day there are quite a number of New-Church clergymen, in this country and England, and a large number of laymen, who, after a careful examination of the subject, are satisfied that the good wine of the Word and the Writings, and the only wine suitable for use as a Communion wine, is always the fruit of the vine, and never fermented wine. Many of these clergymen and church members have not always thought thus, and did not when I commenced writing upon the subject.

At the Annual Meetings of the General Convention of the New Church, when unfermented as well as fermented wine has been permitted to be used, and full notice has been given, nearly or quite one-third of the members present have deliberately partaken of unfermented wine.

I am satisfied, from what I have seen and heard, that one of the most useful works which the Lord has enabled me to do was the writing and sending the reply to "Communion Wine" to over 80,000 clergymen. The clergy of the prevailing organizations are not so difficult to reach upon this subject as are a majority of those of the New Church, for they have not confirmed themselves in favor of fermented wine from the writings for the New Dispensation. It is one thing to see new truths when they are revealed, but it is another step to be willing to see that those truths condemn falses in which we have strongly confirmed ourselves, or evil habits in which we delight, and to avoid confirming ourselves in falses, and to avoid striving to justify evils. To do the latter means to endure and resist temptations, and to engage in a warfare until the old man with his deeds is put off.

The New Church is descending from God out of heaven, and as it progresses, fermented wine is disappearing from the Communion tables of Christian Churches.

"The new wine," says Swedenborg, "is the Divine Truth of the New Testament, and thus of the New Church." (A. R. 316.)

The new wine for the New Christian Church is unfermented wine, pure as it comes from the hands of our Lord and Saviour, Jesus Christ, in the fruit of the vine, and not a leavened wine. And when men return to its exclusive use, multitudes now enslaved, diseased, and insane from leavened wine will be set free, cured and restored to their right mind by the Great Physician—by the inflowing life from Him through this physical representative of His blood.

The New Church is not a new sect or organization, but a new faith and a renewed life resulting from a revelation of Divine Truth, made by the Lord through Emanuel Swedenborg, for the benefit of all sects and all men, that the Christian Church may "revive again" and be reunited in the bonds of Charity, by worshiping the one God whose name is one—even the Lord Jesus Christ—and by striving to live a life according to His commandments.

CHAPTER X.

FINAL APPEAL TO THE CLERGY.

I again appeal to you, as Christian men, to lay aside prejudice and preconceived ideas, if you are troubled with any that have come down to you from darker ages, and to patiently examine the writings of Emanuel Swedenborg.

If you desire and are prepared to read with open eyes and a willing heart, you can but see that the fig-tree is putting forth its leaves, and that we are living in the dawning light and warmth of a new summer. Look at the radical changes which have taken place within the last one hundred and thirty-five years, and are taking place to-day with increasing rapidity, in every department of science, arts, mechanics, medicine, and even in the religious sentiments of the people and in theology, and in civil and ecclesiastical governments, and you may rest assured, that as certain as the Word of the Lord is true, so sure it is that we are now seeing but the beginning of the changes which are yet to be witnessed; for the sure word of prophecy is, "Behold, I make all things new"—New Heavens and a New Earth—old things are to pass away, and we can see that they are passing away.

Swedenborg assures us that he was permitted by the Lord to witness the Last Judgment in 1757, which, like all general judgments, took place in the spiritual world. The Lord when on earth declared, "Now is the judgment of this world, now is the prince of this world cast out. " Swedenborg tells us that between the Lord's first coming and His second coming vast societies were organized in the world of spirits, which is intermediate between heaven and hell, from among those who were not fully prepared for either heaven or hell; and they were associated with those of like affections and persuasions in this world. As the First Christian Church became gradually perverted by false doctrines and evils of life, and as its members increased in the spiritual world, their influence was more and more felt among the religious societies in this world, interfering with the inflowing of good and truth from the Lord and His Word into the minds of men, and threatening their ability to see and obey the truth. The judgment consisted in a new influx of Divine truth into such societies, the effects of which were such that those who were really good were received into heaven, and those who were evil joined their like in hell, glad to escape from the new inflowing of heavenly light and life. In this way they were separated from men on the earth and human freedom reestablished. The effects of that judgment are today gradually being manifested here on earth.

Swedenborg tells us that he witnessed the downfall of Babylon the great in the spiritual world. By Babylon is meant those who are in the love of spiritual dominion over the souls of men. And also he witnessed the casting down of the Dragon. By the Dragon is meant those who are in the doctrine of salvation by faith and ceremonials alone.

As the above vast organizations in the spiritual world were then removed from contact with men, I will let Swedenborg speak of some of the results which followed that judgment in the spiritual world, and of those which are following and which must follow in the Church on earth.

"After the Last Judgment (in 1757) a new heaven was formed from among Christians, only from those, however, who acknowledged the Lord to be the God of heaven and earth, and also repented in the world of their evil works. From this heaven the New Church on earth, which is the New Jerusalem, descends, and will continue to descend.... And the New Church on earth makes one with the New Heaven." (Preface to A. R.)

"In this new Christian heaven are all those who, from the first formation of the Christian Church, worshiped the Lord and lived according to His commandments in the Word, and were therefore in charity and faith from the Lord through the Word." (A. R. 876.)

Swedenborg tells us that "the slavery and captivity in which the man of the Church was formerly" were removed by the Last Judgment; so that "he can now, from restored liberty, more easily perceive interior truths if he has a desire for them." (L. J. 74.) And again he tells us that, as a result of the Last Judgment, the people of Christendom "would be in a more free state of thinking on matters of faith, that is, on spiritual things which relate to heaven, because spiritual liberty has been restored to them" (L. J. 73); and that consequently "the state of the world and of the Church before the Last Judgment," compared with what it was, or was to be after, "was as evening and night compared with morning and day." (Contin. L. J.)

Personal Experience of a Physician

Now can we not all see that the very changes anticipated in the above quotations are rapidly taking place in the Christian world all around us? Men and women are beginning to cease to be willing to be led blindly by clergymen and creeds, with their understandings under subjection to dogma. Many of our clergy, we see, are not willing to be thus led. Swedenborg tells us that in this New Dispensation men are to be led in freedom according to reason, and that professing to believe doctrines which they neither understand nor perceive to be true is of very little use to men.

As false doctrines are passing away, is it not of vast moment that true and rational doctrines should take their place, that our houses and churches be not left desolate? Somewhat extensively among the clergy, and far more extensively among scientists and intelligent people, is the Divine origin of the Sacred Scriptures being called in question. In the writings of Swedenborg, as has already been stated, you will find this question clearly and distinctly settled, for you are there shown that they are written according to the law of correspondence between natural and spiritual things, and therefore that they contain a connected spiritual sense which causes them to differ from all merely human writings, and demonstrates their Divine origin to all who are willing to examine and to see the truth. The day is not far distant when, in the Christian Church, the Sacred Scriptures will be reverenced as they have never been before; for the coming of the Son of Man in the Clouds of Heaven, or in the literal sense of the Word, is with power and great glory.

Even now in the dawning light old false doctrines are rapidly passing away. Look! What congregation would be willing to sit quietly and hear the doctrine of infant damnation proclaimed? Who is satisfied with the doctrine of election and predestination as taught but a few years ago? That favorite doctrine of my childhood's days, the vicarious atonement as taught then, is trembling in the balance, for it is being found not to accord with the Word of the Lord, nor does it appeal to human reason. The doctrine of a trinity of Divine Persons will soon follow. How few even now believe in the resurrection of the material body! Our church members are rapidly coming to believe with St. Paul that there is a natural body and there is a spiritual body, and that the spiritual body is raised at death, and that flesh and blood cannot inherit the Kingdom of God. The doctrine of a literal hell of fire and brimstone, as taught but a few years ago, is rarely taught to-day.

And now, Christian ministers, as these old doctrines are departing, what have you to substitute for them? You know very well that when extreme views are given up, there is great danger that opposite extreme views will be substituted.

Troublesome questions are arising to-day before the clergy and in our churches, which require to be handled with care by intelligent and wise men, if the Lord and His Word are to be reverenced in our churches as they should be, and men are to be led to live heavenly lives.

The question of probation after death is troubling many clergymen and laymen at this day. They see that men and women often leave this world in a very uncertain state of life, so far as they can judge, ill prepared for either heaven or hell; what is to-become of them is the question. Are they all to put away their false doctrines and evils of life and go to heaven, as some believe; or are some of them to go through purgatory and finally, after being purified, to enter heaven, and the rest go to hell, as others believe? Or again, has a man the same chance of choosing and the same ability to choose between truth and falsehood and good and evil, and of shaping his life there, as he has here?

Upon these questions the New Revelations made by the Lord through Emanuel Swedenborg throw a flood of rational light. They show us that heaven is not a place into which a man can be let as a matter of favor; but that, for a man to enter heaven, heaven must be within him. Heaven consists in loving supremely the Lord and the neighbor, or obedience to the Divine Commandments. Hell consists in loving self, money, vain show, ruling over others without regard to use, or sensual gratifications supremely. Before a man can become a resident of hell, hell must be within him. Men enter the other world in much the same state as they leave this world; death does not change their essential characters. Good angels appointed by the Lord strive to teach heavenly truths to all, and to lead all into heavenly affections and societies who are willing to be led. But as the Lord respects the freedom of all men in this world and compels no man to love Him, his neighbor, or obedience to the Divine Commandments supremely, He compels no man there. The Lord casts no one into hell, but when our material bodies are put off and we appear among the inhabitants of the spiritual world, our thoughts and intentions can be seen more clearly than in this world; consequently the good and evil necessarily separate; and finally every one sooner or later associates with his like, the good forming heavenly societies and the evil, infernal societies.

It is evident that those who are guided in all they think and do by either love of the Lord, the neighbor, or of obeying the Divine Commandments, need no penal laws or punishments. It is equally evident that men who are actuated by the supreme love of self, vain show, or sensual gratifications must be restrained, in that world as in this, by penal laws and punishments. But we are told that the Lord governs the hells as well as the heavens through His angels, and does not permit vindictive or unjust punishments. All punishments in that world are reformatory, or for the purpose of restraining spirits from evil doing, and protecting others, as all punishments should be in this world. The Lord's tender mercies are around all His creatures in that world as well as in this, and He strives to make all happy. Even the evil man is permitted to enjoy his delight so long as he does not interfere with or harm others or himself.

Here in this state of probation good and evil men dwell together in the same society, so that the evil have good instruction and good examples, and every chance for repentance and reformation; but in hell they dwell among their like, and it would seem that they are not so favorably circumstanced for changing their life's love there as in this world. In the world of spirits into which we enter at death, all who are not fully prepared by their lives here for heaven or hell tarry until their characters are fully developed, when each one goes to his own congenial society either in heaven or hell, according to his ruling love.

Swedenborg, so far as he was permitted, describes what he saw in the spiritual world; but he did not claim to be a prophet—the future, he tells us, is known to the Lord alone, not even to the angels. Some of the readers of his writings, from certain passages contained therein, have come to think that the Lord in His loving kindness may yet so change the inhabitants of hell that they may be received into heavenly societies, as some have drawn from the letter of the Sacred Scriptures a similar conclusion; while a majority of readers, in both cases, have come to a different conclusion. But the future is known to the Lord alone, and He is love itself, and in His hands we may safely leave the inhabitants of hell; especially as our belief one way or the other will not change the final destiny of a single individual one iota; therefore it is not a practical question.

PREVAILING EVILS OF LIFE.

We are living in the midst of prevailing evils of life which should command the special attention of every clergyman and every Christian. Even infants and children are dying on all sides, and those that survive are being contaminated often even in our churches by the example of clergymen and prominent members.

But yesterday, as I was speaking to a very intelligent, well-known citizen of New York, he expressed to me the opinion that gambling and a desire to obtain money or valuables without returning a due equivalent, by purchasing lottery or chance tickets and stock gambling, is a greater evil than selling and drinking intoxicating drinks; and he most earnestly blamed many of our clergy and churches for the prevalence of this great evil; for, as is well known, it is at church fairs that the young and even children frequently take their first lessons, enticed thereto by the hope that they may be able to obtain an article of much value for a trifling sum. In this the work of demoralization commences, and leads naturally to gambling for money, betting on games, horse-racing, buying lottery tickets, and stock gambling, stimulated by the hope of making fortunes by risking small amounts, not stopping to think that what they gain, if successful, others must lose who are probably no better able to lose than they are. How much short of stealing is this? Look at the sad results which follow the practice started in so many of our churches—the poverty, the thieving, the failures, the breaches of trust, the disgrace and loss of character, and the poor wretches in prison, and others who merit punishment. Christian ministers, is not this a most fearful evil which you, if guilty of encouraging it, should put away from your own lives and teach your people to shun as a sin against God?

Again, it is the duty of husbands and wives to reproduce their species or to multiply and replenish the earth, and this is the most important use of life. Yet a vast multitude of women, by tight dressing to gratify vanity, impair health and their ability to bear healthy, well-formed children, and even their ability to nurse such as are born to them; and such deformed women walk into and out of our churches as examples to young girls, without one word of admonition. And some church members deliberately shirk the responsibility of rearing families of children, either because it is not fashionable to have large families, or because children would interfere with their selfish or sensual enjoyment; and this is not the worst which could be said of some.

Now, although it is equally the duty of all husbands and wives to multiply and replenish the earth, yet church members who, either for the want of ability or inclination, have no children, and bachelors and maidens who do not marry, will stand idly by and see the husbands and wives, however poor they may be, who are willing to do their duty, take the entire care of their children until they reach adult age; they deliberately leave the entire responsibility upon the parents of caring for and raising the money required for the support of the children, who are to be the men and women of the next generation. Is this right? It is true that public schools have been established, for all feel that it will not be safe for the children, who are to rule our country a few years hence to grow up in ignorance.

Men and women will roll in their thousands and hundreds of thousands and even millions, and see the toiling, struggling, hardworking brothers and sisters, sometimes even in the same church organization, striving to do faithfully their part in the care of the children who are to people and replenish the earth, without feeling that they have any responsibility or duty to perform in the way of giving a helping hand in this most important work of life. Now I ask you, brethren of the Christian Church, are such things in accordance with the grand and noble precepts of Christianity, in which we profess to believe—thou shalt love thy neighbor as thyself? Of course, husbands and wives who are able are but too glad to take care of their own children; but there are multitudes who need help. If wealthy husbands and wives are not willing or able to have children, or if bachelors and maidens are not willing to marry and have children, have they no duty to perform toward aiding, even financially, and by their own hands if such help is needed, those who do this most important work, and thus add to the number of intelligent and Christian inhabitants of our country? for the want of whom our country is being flooded by multitudes of the most ignorant of other nations, who have comparatively no knowledge of our free institutions and of religious freedom.

It is true that our poorhouses are established at the expense of the public, to which parents who are without means or employment or adequate wages to support their children can go with their children to avoid starvation; but what parents desire to take their children to such institutions? And we have also charitable institutions to which children can be sent to prevent their starving and going naked; but what father or mother likes to part with their children? It is not charity that such need, but the kind, helping hands of Christian brothers and sisters. All things are to be made new. As the light and especially the heat or love of the New Jerusalem descend into the minds of men, hard-hearted selfishness will disappear, and true Christians will love and strive to help one another and all men as they may need.

And now, in conclusion, I appeal to you, Christian ministers, one and all, to diligently read the Revelations made by the Lord at His second coming through His chosen servant, Emanuel Swedenborg, for they will give you new light and, if you are willing, new life. The light is spreading from the East even unto the West, and the day is not far distant when a clergyman, to be acceptable to an intelligent Christian congregation, must be familiar with the grand and rational doctrines and precepts revealed by the Lord for the benefit of the men of our day and the Church of the future.

It must be evident to you even now that many of the clergy and intelligent laymen are steadily drifting in one of two directions; either to a distinct recognition of the Supreme Divinity of the Lord Jesus Christ, of the holiness and Divinity of the Sacred Scriptures and of the life of charity or of obedience to the Divine Commandments as the only way of salvation; or to an ignoring the existence of a personal God, and of course of all revelation from God. There is no middle ground. Choose ye this day whom ye will serve.

Below you will find a notice of a work on the Science of Correspondences, the science in accordance with which all material things were created and the Sacred Scriptures were written. Send for it. It will give you new light.

ADDENDUM.

A REVIEW OF AN ARTICLE ENTITLED "CHRIST AND THE TEMPERANCE QUESTION" IN "THE CHRISTIAN UNION."

In the *Christian Union* for July 11, 1891, will be found an article written by a clergyman which should not be allowed to go unnoticed. The reverend gentleman assumes in that article that "the life and teaching of Jesus Christ constitute a Divine standard for all His followers." And so do I most unequivocally; but I also claim that we should not be blinded by either strong confirmations or sensual appetites in favor of false views and evil habits, so that, having eyes, we see not the truth and consequently cannot lead a life in accordance with the truth. The writer truly says: "Christ is not to be blindly, but intelligently, followed." In other words, I would say the light afforded by science, by well-known facts and ancient history, must be allowed to shine upon such an important question as the one under consideration. Then again, the testimony of distinguished scholars who have devoted years to a careful consideration of the wine question in the light of the Hebrew and Greek Scriptures, of ancient history and science, should not be ignored, and statements made which have repeatedly been shown to have no foundation in truth, but which are contradicted by facts which at this day should be known by every man who attempts to write upon such an important question.

In the consideration of this question the above writer appears to utterly confound good and truth with the evil and false, which, it is manifest, should never be done. His whole argument is based upon assumptions which we shall find, the more carefully we examine them, have no foundation in truth. He assumes that fermented wine is a good and useful article to be used as a beverage, and, after admitting that he thinks the law of Christian love requires a general abstinence at the present day, he says: —

"But I trust that this necessity belongs simply to the present epoch, and I am not without hope that we shall yet come to a time—though not in my day—when a pure wine can be used by society with no more seriously evil results than now are produced by the use of tea and coffee."

By pure wine he means fermented wine. He apparently thinks that tea and coffee are harmless drinks. Of this more hereafter. Again he says: —

"Any permanent temperance reform, however great emphasis it may lay on a Christian duty of total abstinence, must draw sharply and maintain stoutly the distinction between total abstinence and temperance, between drunkenness and drinking. It must recognize drunkenness to be everywhere and always a sin, drinking to be made so only by the circumstances; temperance to be always and everywhere a duty, total abstinence to be only a means now to be employed for promoting temperance."

Now let us examine this assumption in the light of science, facts, and history.

First. It is known that all the drunkenness in the world up to the sixth century—and history and even the Bible shows us that there was plenty of it, and this the above writer admits—was caused by drinking fermented wine and other fermented drinks, for the art of distillation was unknown. And almost all of the drunkenness in our country at this day results either directly from men and boys drinking wine, beer, or other fermented drinks, or from the appetite thus formed leading them on to the use of distilled liquors; for it is rarely that they commence by using such liquors. There has never been an age in the world's history when the drinking of fermented wine did not lead large numbers of those who drank it to drunkenness, and it is safe to say that in no age of the world has there ever been more drunkenness among those who drink at all than there is at this day.

As to temperance: That old philosopher, Aristotle, tells us that temperance consists in the moderate use of things good and useful, and total abstinence from things injurious.

Second. Fermented wine is either one of the good gifts of God, to be used as a drink to build up and supply the wants of the human body, and may be used freely as we may use milk, the unfermented juice of grapes, and water, or it is not. Let us examine this question carefully for a few moments. We all know that there are animal, vegetable, and mineral substances which act as poisons when taken into the stomach, and that to thus use them is to violate the laws of health and life and to seriously endanger health, reason, and life; and not a few are destroyed by their use. The Divine commandment in regard to all such we know is, "Thou shall not" use them if they kill or endanger life when used. We know that there are other substances which are useful and necessary to nourish and build up the body and give it strength and health. How are we to distinguish these two classes of substances? By their effects on the body we may distinguish between good and useful substances and poisons. There is a natural appetite for wholesome food, which is satisfied by the usual quantity, and the middle-aged and old do not require any more nor even as much as the young man. But for poisons, unless they are made sweet by other substances, there is no natural appetite, but it has to be cultivated by using the poison; but when the appetite is once developed no other substance in nature will satisfy the appetite for it, and the appetite demands that the quantity taken shall be steadily increased to relieve the craving and diseased symptoms which the poison has caused; and if the natural inclination to increase the quantity or frequency is followed, unrestrained by caution or conscience, the individual comes at last to be able to take a quantity with impunity which would kill more than one person not addicted to its use. We all know that this is notably true in regard to fermented wine and other alcoholic drinks, opium and tobacco.

Again, all poisons, when taken into the stomach in a sufficient quantity and length of time, cause specific diseases characteristic of the poison taken. Healthy food does not do this. You see a man reeling in the streets, or drunk on the sidewalk, or with rum-blossoms on his face; you know that he has been drinking fermented wine or some fluid containing its chief ingredient—alcohol. Now, unfermented wine and other healthy drinks never cause such specific diseases or symptoms, however freely used.

Here then, in the characteristics given above, is a broad gulf, as broad and deep as that between Heaven and Hell, between nourishing, life-giving substances and the poisons named above. Of the one we are to use temperately, but from the latter we are to totally abstain. "Thou shalt not" is clearly written.

In all ages fermented wine has been regarded as a poison. In the Bible it is likened to the poison of dragons and the cruel venom of asps. Solomon tells us not to look upon it, for at last it biteth like a serpent and stingeth like an adder. Clement of Alexandria, who lived at the close of the second century, says: "From its use arise excessive desires and licentious conduct. The circulation is accelerated, and the body inflames the soul. "—*Divine Law as to Wines*.

We know by observation that fermented wine is a fluid which fills man when he drinks of it as freely as he may of healthy needed drinks with all manner of uncleanness of both body and soul. How can a clergyman talk of using such a fluid temperately? Can we steal temperately, bear false witness temperately, commit adultery temperately, or murder temperately? Is it right to deliberately do any of these acts temperately? If it is, then it is right to deliberately drink fermented wine temperately, which we know endangers health, freedom, reason and life, and leads men to commit crimes even the most filthy. One glass leads naturally to another, and that to many; just as stealing pennies leads to stealing dollars, and hundreds and thousands of dollars. A perverted appetite or passion can never be fully satisfied, but it leads to sorrow. All such evils must be shunned totally as sins against God.

It would be difficult to find elsewhere in the English language, in so few lines, as many statements so absolutely untrue, dogmatically proclaimed, as in the following from the article in the *Christian Union*: —

"This notion of two wines, one fermented, the other unfermented, must be dismissed as a pure invention, unsupported by any facts, unsanctioned by any scholarship. There was but one wine known to the ancients—fermented grape-juice. This was the wine Christ made, drank, blessed. There was no other used in His time or known to His day."

First, as to scholarship. Does the writer of the above believe that he is superior as to scholarship to the following distinguished scholars, all of whom believe in "this notion of two wines, one fermented and the other unfermented, " several of whom, after a most patient and careful examination of the question, have written one or more volumes upon the subject, and one of them has been twice to the Bible lands for the purpose of carefully investigating the question there and verifying his statements? viz., Moses Stuart, Eliphalet Nott, Alonzo Potter, George Bush, Albert Barns, William M. Jacobus, Taylor Lewis, Geo. W. Sampson, Leon C. Field, F. R. Lees, Norman Kerr, Canon Farrar, Canon Wilberforce, Dawson Burns, Wm. Ritchie, George Duffield, C. H. Fowler, Wm. Patton, Adam Clarke, J. M. Van Buren, S. M. Isaacs, Wm. M. Thayer, John J. Owen; Charles Hartwell, and many other writers I could name, who, after a most critical examination of the question, have written earnestly in favor of the "notion of two wines, one fermented and the other unfermented. " In view of the opinion of such men as these, can the above writer say truthfully that the "notion of two wines" is "unsanctioned by any scholarship"? Have we any more distinguished scholars than those I have named? Are not scholars who have for years made a special study of a question like this, in all of its aspects, much more competent to judge correctly than those who have not? It is certain that the writer in the *Christian Union* has never examined both sides of this question with the slightest care; for if he had done so, as an honest Christian man, as I trust he is, he could never have made many of the statements he has made. He says that the "notion of two wines" is unsupported by any facts, and that "there was but one kind of wine known to the ancients—fermented grape-juice. " Has he never read the Bible—even the New Testament? I shall first bring the testimony of the Lord Himself against him. He says: —

"Neither do men put new wine (*oinon neon*) into old bottles; else the bottles break, and the wine runneth out, and the bottles perish; but they put new wine into new bottles, and both are preserved. " Matt, ix, 17.

Here we have the fresh, unfermented juice of the grape called wine—"new wine. " It could not be put into old bottles and be preserved, for old bottles, especially skin bottles, are sure to contain leaven cells, which would inevitably cause fermentation and burst the bottles, whether they were of skins, glass, or earthenware. We know that fermented wine can be preserved in old bottles, and that it is so preserved without bursting the bottles. Here, then, the fresh, unfermented juice of grapes is called wine by the Lord. Should not our clergy heed His testimony?

There is no difficulty in preserving the juice of grapes, or new wine, unfermented by various methods described by ancient writers. Thus Columella, who lived during the Apostolic days, tells us to fill bottles with fresh grape-juice and seal or cork them carefully and sink them in a well of cold water and fermentation will not ensue. I have tried it successfully; any one can do the same. Next, fill a new or clean bottle with new wine just pressed from the grapes up to its neck, then pour about half an inch of sweet oil on the surface of the wine and cork it carefully, leaving a little space between the cork and oil, and stand the bottle in a cellar, and it will keep. I have three bottles thus preserved free from fermentation for over three years; the cork must not be removed and the bottle must not be shaken. Again, heat the juice to 185 [degrees] Fahr., or to the boiling-point if you please, bottle, cork, and seal it, and it will never ferment.

Now we will turn hastily to the Old Testament. In Isaiah xvi, 10, we read: "The treaders shall tread out no wine (*yayin*) in their presses. " Here we have the juice of grapes, as it is trodden from grapes, called wine.

In Jeremiah xl, 10, 12, we read: "But gather ye wine (*yayin*) and summer fruits and oils, " and we read that they "gathered wine and summer fruits very much. " Here we have the juice of grapes called wine, as it is gathered in with other fruits.

Chapter xlviii, 33: "And I have caused wine (*yayin*) to fail from the wine-presses. "

Dr. Adam Clarke says: "The Hebrew, Greek, and Latin words which are rendered 'wine' mean simply the expressed juice of the grape. "

This juice, like our cider, may be fermented or unfermented, and it is still called by the same name. Here, then, in both the New and Old Testaments, we have the unfermented juice of grapes distinctly recognized as wine, and called wine; and all admit that the fermented juice of grapes is called wine, consequently there are two wines. And distinguished scholars say: —

"In all the passages where the good wine is named (in the Bible), there is no lisp of warning, no intimation of danger, no hint of disapprobation, but always of decided approval. How bold and strongly marked is the contrast!

"The *one* the cause of intoxication, of violence, and of woes; "The *other* the occasion of comfort and of peace. "The *one* the cause of irreligion and of self-destruction; "The *other* the devout offering of piety on the altar of God. "The *one* the symbol of the divine wrath; "The *other* the symbol of spiritual blessings. "The *one* the emblem of eternal damnation; "The *other* the emblem of eternal salvation. " — *Bible Wines*.

"The *one* the cause of intoxication, of violence, and of woes;
"The *other* the occasion of comfort and of peace.

Personal Experience of a Physician

"The *one* the cause of irreligion and of self-destruction;
"The *other* the devout offering of piety on the altar of God.
"The *one* the symbol of the divine wrath;
"The *other* the symbol of spiritual blessings.
"The *one* the emblem of eternal damnation;
"The *other* the emblem of eternal salvation. "—*Bible Wines*.

"The distinction in *quality* between the good and the bad wine is as clear as that between good and bad men, or good and bad wives, or good and bad spirits; for one is the constant subject of warning, designated poison literally, analogically, and figuratively; while the other is commended as refreshing and innocent, which no alcoholic wine is. "—*Lees' Appendix*, p. 232.

Tirosh is another Hebrew word that is often used in the Old Testament for grapes and the juice of grapes, like our word must, but it is rarely if ever applied to the juice after fermentation has commenced. We read: "They shall gather together corn and new wine (*tirosh*), they shall eat together and praise Jehovah, and *they who are gathered together shall drink it in the courts of my holiness.* "—Isaiah lxii, 9.

And again, in regard to *tirosh*, we read: "That thou mayest gather in thy corn, thy wine (*tirosh*), and thine oil. " (Deut. xi, 14.) "Thus saith the Lord, as the new wine (*tirosh*) is found in the cluster, and *one* saith destroy it not, for a blessing is in it. " (Isaiah lxv, 8.) "And thou shalt eat before the Lord thy God in the place He shall choose, the tithe of thy corn and wine (*tirosh*). " (Deut. xiv, 22.) Here we see that *tirosh* was to be eaten.

The word *tirosh* occurs thirty-eight times in the Hebrew Bible.

It is translated into Greek, in the Septuagint, by [seventy] distinguished Hebrew scholars, about three centuries before the Christian era, as follows: "The LXX renders *tirosh* in every case but two by *oinos* (the Greek word for wine), the generic name for *yayin*. "

Now, are we for a moment to suppose that the above seventy distinguished ancient scholars did not understand as well what was included under the name of wine in their day, as does the writer in the *Christian Union* to-day, when they classed the unfermented juice of grapes with wine, and called it wine? How can the above writer say that "there was but one kind of wine known to the ancients—

fermented grape juice"? Unfermented wine not known to the ancients, indeed! How utterly contrary to the truth, and to well-known facts, is such a statement. Just look a moment, gentle reader—

"Aristotle ('Meteorologica, ' iv, 9) says of the sweet wine of his day ([Greek Text]), that it did not intoxicate ([Greek Text]). And Athenaeus ('Banquet, ' ii, 24) makes a similar statement. "—*Oinos.*

"Josephus, the Jewish historian, paraphrasing the dream of Pharaoh's butler, who dreamed that he took clusters of grapes and pressed them into Pharaoh's cup, and gave the cup to Pharaoh, repeatedly calls this grape-juice *wine.* Bishop Lowth, 1778, in his 'Commentary' (Isaiah v, 2) says: 'The fresh juice pressed from the grape' was by Herodotus styled *oinos ampelinos*, that is, wine of the vine. "—*Wine of the Word.*

The celebrated Opimian wine, which Pliny [born A. D. 23] tells us (xiv, 4) had in his day, two centuries after it was made, the consistency of honey, was unquestionably an inspissated article. Such was the Taeniotic wine of Egypt, which Athenaeus, in his "Banquet" (i, 25), tells us had such a degree of richness that "it is dissolved little by little when it is mixed with water, just as the Attic honey is dissolved by the same process. "

"There is abundance of evidence, " says the Rev. Dr. Patton, "that the ancients mixed their wines with water; not because they were so strong with alcohol as to require dilution, but because, being rich syrups, they needed water to prepare them for drinking. The quantity of water was regulated by the richness of the wine and the time of year. "

"Aristotle (born about B. C. 384) testifies that the *wines of Arcadia* were so thick that they dried up in goat-skins, and that it was the practice to scrape them off and dissolve the scrapings in water. " (Meteorology, iv, 10.)—"Temperance Bible Commentary. "

We know very well that these ancient wines, which were called wine in those days, which did not intoxicate, and others that were as thick as honey, were not fermented wines; for fermented wines do intoxicate, and wines as thick as honey cannot be made from fermented wine, for the albuminous and other substances which make condensed wines thick are cast down or out, or destroyed by fermentation. I have four samples of such condensed wines, or grape-juice, which are as thick as honey. One I obtained at Buda-Pesth, Hungary; one in Cairo, Egypt; one in Damascus, Asia; and the fourth was condensed and sent to me by a gentleman then residing in California. I have had these samples now over six years.

Why should the writer in the *Christian Union* quote from another writer, and thus try to make it appear that the ancient condensed wines were nothing but "grape jellies"? Does he not know that they are very different preparations, and prepared by different methods? Condensed wines are prepared by crushing and pressing the juice from the pulp, skins, and seeds, and then boiling or otherwise evaporating the water until the juice is as thick as honey, so that it can be easily preserved from fermentation? whereas grape jellies are made by boiling the grapes until they are well cooked, then rubbing or squeezing all the pulp and skins practicable through a colander, sieve, or coarsely-woven strainer; and then sugar is added to sweeten and aid in forming a jelly. Condensed wines will dissolve in water as we are told the ancient thick wines did, but grape jellies will do so only very imperfectly, for they are composed largely of the pulp of the grape.

The writer in the *Christian Union* tells us, in a passage already quoted, speaking of fermented wine: —

"This was the wine Christ made, drank, blessed."

And again he says: —

"He (Christ) commenced His public ministry by making, by a miracle, wine in considerable quantity, and this apparently only to add to the joyous festivities of a wedding. He apparently used wine customarily, if not habitually. When He was about to die, He chose wine as the symbol of His blood, shed for many for the remission of sins, asked His Father's blessing on a cup containing wine, passed it to His disciples with the direction, 'Drink ye all of it.'"

Now, intelligent Christian reader, what are we to think of the above statements? Let us look at these statements in the light of reason, common sense, science, and revelation. Is it probable, is it possible, that at that wedding feast, after the guests had drank freely of an intoxicating wine, that our blessed Lord, guided by love and wisdom, would create a large quantity more of an intoxicating wine for them to drink? It is not possible; and the assumption is flatly contradicted by the Governor of the feast, who pronounced the wine created as the "best wine. " Place to the lips of a child of parents who do not use intoxicating drinks, or to a man or woman who never drinks such drinks, two glasses, one containing a well-fermented wine, and the other containing the sweet, delicious juice of good ripe grapes, and there is not the slightest doubt as to which would be chosen and pronounced "best" every time—try it.

Then again, is it possible that, on that occasion, a kind of wine was made of which the Lord has never created a single drop in the fruit of the vine? Fermented wine is a product of leaven or ferment and of man's ingenuity; and its chief and essential constituent, alcohol, for which men drink it, is an effete product, and holds a similar relation to the leaven that urine does to the animal body. As Pasteur says, "ferment eats, as it were, " or consumes the nourishing and useful ingredients in the juice of the grapes, decomposes them, and casts out excretions, as man does when he eats grapes. Consequently, fermented wine is an utterly unclean fluid, and it fills man, when he drinks it, with all manner of uncleanness, mentally and physically, from the crown of his head to the soles of his feet, as we well know. It is preeminently a leavened substance, for it is never purified by heat, as is leavened bread. We have an abundance of testimony, which the reverend writer of the article ignores, that the Orthodox Jews have regarded, in all ages, and do to-day as a rule regard, fermented wine as coming under the restrictions placed upon leavened things.

The celebrated Jewish Rabbi, S. M. Isaacs, said in 1869: "The Jews do not use in their feasts for sacred purposes fermented drinks of any kind. The marriage feast is a sacrament with us. "

In a recent work (1879) written by a Jewish Rabbi, the Rev. E. M. Myers, entitled "The Jews, their Customs and Ceremonies, with a full account of all their Religious Observances from the Cradle to the Grave, " we read that among the strictly orthodox Jews, "During the entire festival (of the Passover) no leavened food nor fermented liquors are permitted to be used, in accordance with Scriptural injunctions. " (Ex. xii, 15, 19, 20; Deut. xvii, 3, 4.) This, we think, settles the question so far as the Orthodox Jews are concerned; and their customs, without much question, represent those prevailing at the time of our Lord's advent.

Personal Experience of a Physician

The editor of the London *Methodist Times* lately witnessed the celebration of the Jewish Passover in that city, and at the close of the services said to the Rabbi: "May I ask with what *kind* of wine you have celebrated the Passover this evening? " The answer promptly given was: —

"With a non-intoxicating wine. Jews never use fermented wine in their synagogue services, and must not use it on the Passover, either for synagogue or home purposes. Fermented liquor of any kind comes under the category of 'leaven, ' which is proscribed in so many well-known places in the Old Testament. * * * I have recently read the passage in Matthew in which the Paschal Supper is described. There can be no doubt whatever that the wine used upon that occasion was unfermented. Jesus, as an observant Jew, would not only not have drunk fermented wine on the Passover, but would not have celebrated the Passover in any house from which everything fermented had not been removed. I may mention that the wine I use in the service at the synagogue is an infusion of raisins. You will allow me, perhaps, to express my surprise that Christians, who profess to be followers of Jesus of Nazareth, can take what He could not possibly have taken as a Jew—intoxicating wine—at so sacred a service as the Sacrament of the Lord's Supper. "

It is utterly impossible that Jesus Christ could have used fermented wine as a symbol of His blood, for in its essential constituents, which are alcohol, vinegar, etc., it bears not the slightest resemblance to blood; whereas unfermented wine, in its essential constituents, which are albumen, sugar, etc., bears the greatest resemblance to blood. This simple fact ought to satisfy every intelligent man.

Then again, our Lord, when He took the cup and blessed and said, "Drink ye all of it, " knowing that fermented wine was included under the name of wine, and as if foreseeing that His followers might mistake and use intoxicating wine, carefully avoided the use of the word wine at all, and called it the "fruit of the vine, " which unfermented wine is and fermented wine is not. It does seem that these facts should satisfy every intelligent, Christian man. Can there be, my Christian brethren, a greater profanation of a holy ordinance than the use of the drunkard's cup as a communion wine, instead of the fruit of the vine? By the use of fermented wine as a communion wine many a man who was struggling to reform his life has been led back to drunkenness and death. I have known of some sad instances.

It might be well for some of our clergy to hear and heed the warning voice of the Sacred Scriptures: —

"'It is not for kings to drink wine, nor princes strong drink, lest they drink and forget the law and pervert the judgment of the afflicted.' Here is abstinence enjoined, and the reason for it plainly given. Again (Lev. x, 8-11), *it is required of the priests*: 'And the Lord spake unto Aaron, saying, Do not drink wine nor strong drink, thou, nor thy sons with thee, when ye go into the tabernacle of the congregation, lest ye die: it shall be a statute for ever throughout your generations: That ye may put a difference between holy and unholy, and between unclean and clean; and that ye may teach the children of Israel all the statutes which the Lord hath spoken unto them by the hand of Moses.'"

"Wine is a mocker, strong drink is raging: and whosoever is deceived thereby is not wise."—Prov. xx, i.

No one questions that the wine referred to above as unholy and a mocker and unclean, is fermented wine, and no one supposes for a moment that it is unfermented wine. "But they also have erred through wine, and through strong drink are out of the way; the priest and the prophet have erred through strong drink, they are swallowed up of wine, they are out of the way through strong drink, they err in vision, they stumble in judgment. For all tables are full of vomit and filthiness, so that there is no place clean." (Isa. xxviii, 7,8.)

How correctly and literally do the above words represent the effects of drinking fermented wine and strong drinks, seen today as of old. O gentlemen of the clergy! beware! beware! "Woe to him that giveth his neighbor drink; that putteth thy bottle to him." (Hab. ii, 5,15.) You have young and inexperienced men and women and even boys under your charge. May the Lord protect them!

CANON WILBERFORCE ON SACRAMENTAL WINES.

Canon Wilberforce is reported by the London *Temperance Record* as saying at a recent meeting in England: "He believed if people desired to go back literally and absolutely to the days of the institution of the Sacrament, it would be a most difficult thing, if not impossible, to prove that the particular cup which their Master took in His hand in that solemn crisis of His life when He instituted the Holy Eucharist was fermented at all. There was abundant testimony to prove it was not. Some went back to primitive authorities. He should like to read one or two which might have weight with them. Take for example the testimony of St. Cyprian, who wrote in A. D. 230: —

"'When the Lord gives the name of His body to bread, composed of the union of many particles, He indicates that our people, whose sins He bore, are united. And when He calls wine squeezed out from bunches of grapes His blood, He intimates that our flocks are similarly joined by the varied admixture of a united multitude.'"

"This distinctly implied, for all he knew, squeezing bunches of grapes. But there was more important testimony from one man who was considered by a certain party in the Church of great value—St. Thomas Aquinas, a great father of the 13th century. He said: —

"'The juice of ripe grapes, on the other hand, has already the form of wine; for its sweet taste evidences a mellowing change, which is its completion by natural heat (as it is said in the "Meteorologica," iv, 3, not far from the beginning), and for that reason this Sacrament can be fulfilled by the juice of grapes.'"

While in Egypt in 1884 I visited the American missionaries, and asked them what kind of wine they used as a communion wine in their churches. They told me that almost all of their members were from among the Copts, who are the descendants from the early Christians of Egypt, who have been comparatively isolated and separated from the Christian world for many centuries, and when they told them that the Western Christians used fermented wine, or "shop wine," as they called it, they were horrified at the idea, and would not partake of it; so they steeped or soaked raisins in water, and then pressed the juice from them and used that, as has been done by the Orthodox Jews when they could not obtain pure unfermented wine. I visited the Grand Patriarch of the Coptic Church, and through an interpreter he told me that he did the same, and that it was suitable for use the moment that it was pressed from the raisins. The day is not far distant when the members of the Western Christian churches will be as much horrified at the idea of using fermented wine as a sacramental wine as are the unperverted Christians of Egypt, and this will occur when our clergy and laity cease to be controlled by either strong confirmations or preconceived ideas or by sensual appetites, and can study the Sacred Scriptures and ancient history, and science and well-established facts, in the light of reason and common sense, instead of assuming everything which accords with their desires, and ignoring everything which conflicts therewith.

Again, the writer of the article I am reviewing says: —

"Drunkenness is always and everywhere a sin; whether drinking is a sin depends upon circumstances; and whether the circumstances are such as to make drinking sinful, each individual must decide for himself, and answer for his decision, not to a priesthood, a society, or a newspaper press, but to his own conscience and his God."

While drunk the drunkard is insane, and when not drunk he is an abject slave. His appetite controls him, soul and body; he will sacrifice his property, his reputation, and the comfort of wife and children to gratify it. If, gentle reader, you have witnessed the struggles which some have witnessed of men striving earnestly to break loose from that habit, you would not be so ready to pronounce drunkenness always a sin; you would hardly dare thus to judge the poor victim. God alone can realize what he suffers. I ask the intelligent reader, in the light of reason and common sense and of the Word of God, which is the greater sinner, the man who, after he has witnessed all the wretchedness, sorrows, drunkenness, and deaths which we see around us, deliberately takes his first glass of the fluid which has caused this misery, or continues to drink after he has once commenced, while he has the ability in freedom to restrain his appetite, or the man who, by thus drinking, has lost his freedom and reason, and then drinks to drunkenness? If either is a sinner, can there be any doubt as to which is the greatest sinner? A far greater number, die from steady drinking than from drunkenness; they die from an inability to withstand the ordinary causes of disease, or to resist diseased action when attacked, and vast multitudes die from diseases caused by so-called temperate drinking, short of drunkenness. The statistics of insurance companies show that the average duration of adult human lives is shortened from seventeen to twenty-four per cent. Is it no sin to enter upon or to continue such a life? Is such deliberate self-murder no sin? And again, no man living who commences and continues drinking can have any assurance that he will not become a drunkard. I well remember when a young man, perhaps eighteen years old, standing on my native New England hills, working upon the highway with a young man three or four years older than myself. I said to him that I thought it was well to make up our minds never to drink intoxicating drinks during health, and to join a temperance society;

he differed from me, and he said that when he was tired, or went out in the cold and wet and got chilled, he thought that a little "cider brandy" did him good. "But, " he exclaimed with great energy, "the man who cannot restrain his appetite is a fool! If you ever hear of my getting drunk, tell me, and I will quit drinking. " I intimated to him that it then might be too late. Alas! alas for that young man! he became a drunkard; he spent the farm left by his father; his wife died; his children were scattered among friends; and years after, when I returned to my native town, I was told that he was a pauper at the poorhouse.

We are told by the reverend gentleman in the *Christian Union* that nature produces alcohol in the juices, as though its production was by a natural and orderly process. The process of fermentation is just as natural as the putrefaction of meat, when not prevented by care, and from an altogether similar cause; and as orderly as the eating of grain by rats if no care is taken to prevent it; and it is a no more natural or orderly process. The writer tells us that: —

"Whether the community can properly, without infringing on the liberty of the individual, prohibit all manufacture and sale of alcoholic liquors, is a political question, on which the life and teachings of Christ throw no light. "

A strange statement, indeed! Is it not right to prohibit theft, highway robbery, and other evil acts? Do Christ's teachings throw no light upon such questions? "Thou shall love thy neighbor as thyself. " In our country the government is by the people and for the people, and voters are responsible for the laws made or unmade; and they should be governed by Christ's precepts and not by political cliques. We do not hesitate to enact laws to prohibit druggists and others from selling other well-known poisons to people without the prescription of a physician, for fear they may possibly be used by the purchasers to harm either themselves or others; and I presume the reverend writer does not seriously question the justice and propriety of such laws; yet, strange to say, we license men, and thus give the sanction of the law, to sell fermented wine, beer, and other intoxicating drinks, and allow them to sell tobacco, all deadly poisons, when they know the purchasers will use them to harm themselves and others, and often destroy their lives. Yes, we thus license men to sell when we know that these poisons are sold to men and women who are controlled by an unnatural appetite instead of by reason; when it is known that they have harmed and killed more of the human family than all other poisons put together, and that many of the purchasers, to say the least, will certainly use them to destroy health, reason, and their own lives, and to render their own families and all intimately associated with them unspeakably wretched and unhappy. And yet, exclaims the above writer, whether the community can prohibit such sales of alcoholic liquors or not, without infringing on the liberty of the individual, "is a political question, on which the life and teachings of Christ throw no light. " And the inference is that Christians, preachers, and our religious press have nothing to do with this question. "O consistency! thou art a jewel. " Let stealing become as universal as the selling of intoxicants, and wives and children thereby be deprived of their means of support as extensively as they are by the selling of intoxicants, would the reverend gentleman stand aloof, and represent that the life and teachings of Christ throw no light upon the question of prohibiting such a violation of the Divine commandments? Shall Christians stand aloof from enacting laws to prohibit stealing for fear of infringing on the liberty of individual thieves? Can crimes be prevented without interfering with the "personal liberty" of criminals to commit crimes?

What is stealing when compared to the selling of intoxicating drinks and tobacco as they are sold in our streets, and all over our own and other lands? Kind Christian parents, which in your estimation would be the greatest crime, and which would you prefer, that a thief should steal from your boy or son, before he is twenty-one years of age, or after you cease to be responsible for him, his money, or that a man should sell cigarettes, beer, fermented wine, or other intoxicants unbeknown to you, and take his money, giving these poisons instead, and thus leading him on step by step, until an unnatural appetite is formed, and he becomes a slave to the use of a poison often before he has reached the age when his rational faculties are fully developed; and when by the use of these poisons the full development of his body is prevented, and his prospects for enjoying good health thereafter and of living to the allotted age of man are most materially lessened. In both instances his money is taken, and we know, by the poverty-stricken men and women and young men we see visiting our saloons, that some of the saloonists, as well as the thief, will take his last penny. Which is the greatest crime, to steal a man's money who is under bondage to a perverted appetite, and consequently comparatively irresponsible for his acts, or to sell him the above named poisons, which so seriously prevent development and endanger his health, reason, and life, and which bring such wretchedness and sorrow to so many homes? In both instances the man's money is gone, his wife and children are deprived of the benefit which might result from its legitimate use; but in the one case the man returns to his family a sober, loving husband and father—in the other, perchance, drunk, or on the direct road that leads to drunkenness.

In reply to his intimation that the Bible permits Christians to use fermented wine, but the Koran does not allow Mohammedans to use it, I would simply intimate to the reverend gentleman that the Lord, in His good Providence, has permitted, through the Koran, the Mohammedans to be protected from the drinking of fermented wine and other intoxicating drinks, as He has attempted to protect Christians directly by the numerous warnings in His Word; but the difference lies right here—the former have heeded the warnings, while the latter have not, and hence the fearful drunkenness prevalent in Christian countries. And we see the people of Christian countries sending their whiskey into heathen or Gentile lands with their missionaries. Alas! alas! Which is better—to be a good heathen or a drunken Christian?

A gentleman whom I desired to see resides at Constantinople. He is an Englishman, and when my wife and myself were there in 1885 he had resided there twenty-two years, and had run the largest flouring mill in Turkey. We visited his mill, which was about two miles up the Golden Horn, and he spent an evening with us at the hotel where we were stopping. During our conversation I said to him: "I would like to know about the Mohammedan Turks: what kind of men are they? In our country you can hardly call a man by a worse name than to call him a Turk. " He replied that the Government officials and those who come much in contact with foreigners are apt to be corrupt enough. "But, " he exclaimed with great emphasis, "the laboring Turk! the laboring Turk has a great future before him!! If I want a man to row me down the Golden Horn when the weather is rough, or to watch my mills when I am away and asleep, who I know will do his duty faithfully, I always choose a Turk instead of a Christian. " He admitted that the fact that they never drink fermented wine or other intoxicating drinks was one of the causes of their greater reliability.

"Hon. Chauncey M. Depew will scarcely be accused of fanaticism on the question of liquor drinking. His opinion as a man of wide observation and knowledge of human nature is valuable even to

Personal Experience of a Physician

those who would discount his opinions on the political methods of dealing with the evil. Here is Mr. Depew's experience as stated in a speech before a company of railroad men: —

"'Twenty-five years ago I knew every man, woman, and child in Peekskill. And it has been a study with me to mark boys who started in every grade of life with myself, to see what has become of them. I was up last fall and began to count them over, and it was an instructive exhibit. Some of them became clerks, merchants, manufacturers, lawyers, doctors. *It is remarkable that every one of those that drank is dead;* not one living of my age. Barring a few who were taken off by sickness, *every one who proved a wreck and wrecked his family did it from rum and no other cause.* Of those who were church-going people, who were steady, industrious, and hard-working men, who were frugal and thrifty, every single one of them, without an exception, owns the house in which he lives and has something laid by, the interest on which, with his house, would carry him through many a rainy day. When a man becomes debased with gambling, rum, or drink, he does not care; all his finer feelings are crowded out. The poor women at home are the ones who suffer—suffer in their tenderest emotions; suffer in their affections for those whom they love better than life.'" — *The Voice.*

I think almost every man who is 75 years old, if he will look back and review carefully his youthful acquaintances, can bear almost if not equally as strong testimony as to the effects of intoxicating drinks on human life.

It is certain that but a small proportion of the drinkers who died prematurely were drunkards; they were simply what is called temperate drinkers.

I fully agree with the reverend writer in the *Christian Union* that we should not judge others to be bad or evil men because they do not speak and act just as we think they should, for we cannot see the motives from which their words and acts spring—they are known to the Lord alone; but should we not judge whether a man's words and acts are true and useful and in accordance with the Divine Commandments, or whether they are false and evil and in violation of the commandments? For instance, when we clearly see that the arguments in favor of fermented wine are all based upon assumptions which the most careful investigations by scholars as competent as any in the world show have no foundation in truth, and when we find from historical records that in all ages its use has caused an immense amount of suffering, wretchedness, drunkenness, and an untold number of premature deaths; and we see the same results following its use all around us at this day; and when science teaches us that its use is entirely unnecessary during health, and a direct violation of the laws of health and life; and when in the Sacred Scriptures fermented wine is likened, as to its effects on man, to the poison of dragons and the cruel venom of asps, and Solomon tells us that at last "it biteth like a serpent and stingeth like an adder;"—is it not clearly our duty to show to our fellow-men, and especially to the young, that to commence drinking fermented wine or beer, or to continue to drink so long as we have the power to resist the inclination to drink, is a violation of the commands, Thou shalt not kill, Thou shalt love the Lord thy God supremely, and not the gratification of a perverted appetite; and should we not as clearly as possible point out the truth, and call men to repentance and to the shunning of such evils as sins against God? How else is the world to be reformed and elevated, and the life of the New Jerusalem to descend from God out of heaven, and find an abiding place among men?

The boy, the young man, and those of all ages, in whom the regenerate life has either not commenced or has barely commenced, cannot be expected to live and act up to the Pauline maxim—"if meat cause my brother to offend," etc. Satisfy such that fermented wine is not the "cup of devils," but that it derives its life from the Lord through heaven instead of through hell, and that it is a good and useful drink, and that it is to be hoped the time will come when it can be safely drank, can they want any greater license for commencing and for continuing the life which leads to drunkenness? No one ever intends to become a drunkard or to destroy his life by drinking. He only drinks enough to satisfy his perverted appetite and to make him feel good; that is all.

Now, dear Christian reader, what can be more unfortunate for the Christian Church than for clergymen standing high in the Church, as do several who have written in favor of fermented wine, to write when they possess *only* such an extremely superficial knowledge of the wine question, in its Biblical, historical, scientific, and medical aspects, as is manifested in the article under review, and several others which have been printed and circulated within a few years? And how unfortunate that such articles should ever be published in religious periodicals that enter the homes where dwell children, and the young and innocent as well as drinkers! I thank the Lord that no religious paper bearing such seductive messages ever entered my father's house as I approached manhood.

The greatest obstacle which the grand temperance reformation has to encounter to-day is the stand publicly taken by so many of our clergy and religious periodicals in favor of fermented wine as a good and useful drink, and the use of intoxicating wine as a communion wine in so many of our churches. But the True Light has come into the world, and it will shine more and more until the perfect day.

As to tea and coffee, while they can hardly be compared with intoxicating drinks, tobacco, and opium, as to their injurious effects on man when he uses them, yet they are very far from being harmless; for, like the other poisons named, their use begets an unnatural appetite which healthy fluids will not satisfy, and they cause symptoms and diseases characteristic of the fluid taken. Tea causes sleeplessness, palpitation of the heart, and other symptoms, while coffee causes the "coffee headache, " often destroys the morning appetite; if given to children, interferes with their development, interferes with digestion, and causes a variety of nervous symptoms about the chest and stomach. Parents make a great mistake and do their children great injustice when they allow them to taste of tea or coffee before they are twenty-one years of age, or until they have passed out from their control. If the young can be kept from becoming enslaved by such habits, and consequently remain in freedom, until their rational faculties are fully developed, in the increasing light of this new day, it will not be difficult for them to see that all such substances should be avoided. They do not add to one's enjoyment, for they, like intoxicants, tobacco, and all stimulating condiments, destroy or seriously impair the natural delicacy of taste with which the Lord has endowed us, when we eat or drink wholesome and needed articles of food. I am seventy-six years of age, yet I never had a better appetite, and food never tasted better than it does to-day; and I attribute this to my having so generally avoided improper articles of food and drink. After a most patient and careful examination of both sides of the wine question in the light of Divine Revelation, ancient history and of science, for many years, and after having witnessed the fearful demoralization, the wretchedness and sorrow, the diseases and deaths which result from drinking fermented wine and other intoxicants, nothing so surprises me, and discourages me, in regard to the immediate future of the American people, as the pertinacity and persistency with which so many of the clergy of our country, without any careful examination of both sides of this question, are striving to justify the use of fermented wine as a beverage and even as a Communion wine. Instead of assuming and ignoring everything, let the advocates of fermented wine answer the following inquiry by the Rev. Dr. Eliphalet Nott, President of Union College: "Can the same thing, in the same state, be good and bad; a symbol of wrath and a symbol of mercy; a thing to be sought after and a thing to be avoided? Certainly not. And is the Bible, then, inconsistent with itself? No, certainly."

Printed in the United States
127827LV00006B/60/A